OSTEOPATHIC MECHANICS

A TEXT-BOOK

BY

EDYTHE F. ASHMORE, D. O.

DETROIT

Formerly Professor of Osteopathic Technique,
American School of Osteopathy, Kirksville, Missouri

WITH 82 ILLUSTRATIONS
3 COLORED PLATES

JOURNAL PRINTING CO.

KIRKSVILLE, MISSOURI

1915

PRINTED IN AMERICA
JOURNAL PRINTING COMPANY
KIRKSVILLE, MISSOURI

TO MY MOTHER

EMMA MAGINNIS ASHMORE

WHOSE CONSTANT ENCOURAGEMENT HAS INSPIRED ME TO THE COMPLETION OF THIS WORK

TABLE OF CONTENTS

ERRATA

Page 46, line 22, the words ''lie pon'' should read ''lie upon.''

Page 87, under fig. 35, ''the dottled lines'' should read ''the curved lines.''

Page 88, footnote 2, line 2, the word ''right'' should be inserted between ''thus, a '' and ''rotation lesion.''

Page 97, ''Experimental palpation, E'' should read ''E^2.''

Page 104, line 12, the word ''left'' should replace the word ''right.''

Page 115,, "Experimental palpation, G" should read "G^2".

Page 121, the footnotes should be numbered ''2'' and ''3'' to correspond with the exponent numbers above.

Page 197, line four, ''outward flexion movement'' should read ''outward extension movement.''

Page 199, line 16, should read ''and the normal erect position'' etc.

PREFACE

When Dr. Andrew Taylor Still gave to the world the philosophy of Osteopathy in the establishment of a college for its teaching, the science of Osteopathy was yet in its infancy, for like many of the great sciences, it began as an art in the brain of a master. Thus it is that genius gives to the world that which afterward requires years of careful research and study to confine within the regulations of principle and law. It is not strange, therefore, that in the third decade of the existence of the parent college the first textbook of the mechanics of osteopathy should appear.

The scope of this book is strictly that of a text-book and does not aim to be an exhaustive treatise upon the subject but rather a perspective placing before the mind of the student clearly and briefly certain definite facts with their relative values to the end that he by further study may more easily attain skill in osteopathic diagnosis and practice.

There has been no attempt made at literary brilliancy nor startling originality. I have kept in mind constantly the needs of the student as I have found them in my own college days of fifteen years ago and during the past year while teaching the Junior classes of the American School of Osteopathy. Other writers in our scientific journals have covered well the problems of technique and to them I am much indebted, especially to Drs. Carl P. McConnell and Harry Willis Forbes.

The plan of presentation in this book is distinctly my own for no other teacher to my knowledge has begun the subject of osteopathic mechanics with the study of spinal curvature. From observation I do not hesitate to claim that it has decided merits and in this connection I wish to acknowledge my indebtedness to Robert W. Lovett of Boston whose work "Lateral Spinal Curvature," has enlarged my understanding of the movements of the spine and in a way made possible much of the development of the subject of spinal subluxations.

In the matter of terminology, the larger part of this book was written before the adoption by the American Osteopathic Association of the nomenclature and definitions prepared by a committee of the heads of the department of osteopathic mechanics in the several colleges. Wherever possible I have given both old and new terms.

In the matter of corrective movements, I have endeavored to select the very simplest, those illustrating the principles of correction most plainly. The height of the practitioner, his weight, and physical strength are factors that induce him to modify the leverages he uses in operating osteopathically upon patients who show as many variations from the average type as may the physician himself.

To my students who have helped in the construction of the illustrations of this work I am very grateful and I wish to express here my thanks to Drs. Frances Graves and Anna E. Northup, graduate osteopaths, to Drs. Clifford L. Baker, Oliver C.Foreman, and E. P. Malone of the class of January, 1916, to Miss Beatrice L. Jemmette and Mr. L. P. Riemer of the class of June, 1916, and to Mr. Eugene D. Platt, photographer, of the January, 1917, class.

I desire to express my thanks, also, to the editors of the Journal of Osteopathy for permission to use illustrations that have appeared in their pages and to Dr. Frank P. Millard of Toronto for his kindness in lending me the zinc etchings of the illustrations drawn by himself.

To the Founder of Osteopathy, to whom each osteopath owes all honor and appreciation, I wish to acknowledge the greatest debt of all for the wonderful system of healing which has brought to me and to all others who have been privileged to employ it, the happiness that comes to him or to her who is conscious of having helped to alleviate the suffering of humanity.

EDYTHE F. ASHMORE, D. O.

Kirksville, Mo., July 25, 1915.

OSTEOPATHIC MECHANICS

CHAPTER I.

THE LESION

OSTEOPATHIC MECHANICS is a system of animal mechanics which, taking into consideration the anatomical parts of the human body, especially the bones, ligaments, and muscles, recognizes disturbances in their relations, in particular malalinements and subluxations of joints, and explains the principles by which may be secured the normal apposition and adjustment of part with part. It is embraced by the larger subject of the PRINCIPLES OF OSTEOPATHY, which based upon the sciences of anatomy, chemistry, and physiology, by the application of a distinctive, etiologic, fundamental truth, establishes an exact diagnosis, a clear pathology, and a rational system of therapy.

The central thought of the science of Osteopathy is the lesion, which has been defined as any structural perversion which produces or maintains functional disturbance. The word lesion has been derived from the Latin verb, laedere, to injure. A lesion, then, is any maladjustment which ultimately causes an injury to tissues, or it is an etiological factor in the production of disease and manifests pathological effects. A lesion is itself the result of injury and as such presents certain signs and symptoms. With the production of lesions, with their signs and symptoms, with their removal, are Osteopathic Mechanics concerned. The effects of lesion are covered by the subjects of Osteopathic Pathology and Practice.

The term lesion has been used in a restricted sense to mean any anatomical irregularity of a joint abnormal to the individual and the result of injury originating without the joint and intrinsic or extrinsic to the organism itself. The lesions which produce the most serious effects are those of the spinal articulations, the occiput with the atlas, the sacrum with the fifth lumbar, and the innominates (ossa coxae) with the sacrum, for the reason that these joints are more intimately connected with the two nervous systems, the cranio-spinal and the sympathetic. Joint lesions have been called osseous lesions, for of first consideration in a joint are the articulating surfaces.

Lesions are the result of injury, direct or indirect: direct when acted upon by forces at variance with the usual function of the joint; indirect, when by disturbance in the function of the tissues which maintain the joint in balance, lost equilibrium results. These indirect causes have been termed muscular and ligamentous lesions and should not be confused with the effects manifest in tissues about the joint secondary to osseous maladjustment.

A muscular lesion is a contraction or contracture and is the result of direct violence to the muscle tissue itself or is caused indirectly by disturbance in the nervous mechanism controlling the action of the muscle, from

1. Irritative influences.
    a. Atmospheric changes, heat, cold, etc.
    b. Vaso-motor spasm.
    c. Reflexes from viscera.
    d. Toxins in the blood stream.
    e. Fatigue.
2. Postural defects.
    a. Kyphosis.
    b. Lordosis.
    c. Lateral curvature.
3. Pathological changes in nerve cells or neurons.

A strong contraction or contracture of a muscle brings its origin and insertion closer together and thus may be the first cause of a vertebral osseous lesion.

A ligamentous lesion is one in which there is a changed condition of one or more of the ligaments of the joint; it may be described as a thickening or thinning of the fibrous tissue; it is usually the result of congestion or inflammation and its effects are increased resistance or debility in the joint. Secondarily to ligamentous lesions are found impaction or relaxation osseous lesions.

An impaction lesion of a vertebral articulation is a lesion which is characterized by an approximation of all the bony parts, with a thinning of the intervertebral disc and a thickening of the ligaments about the joint.

A relaxation lesion of a vertebral articulation is a lesion which is characterized by hypermobility, great elasticity of the interarticular fibrocartilage, and a thinning of the ligaments about the joint.

Spinal lesions are named according to the upper of the two vertebræ entering into lesion. A third thoracic lesion means a maladjustment of the third-fourth thoracic articulation. Lesions in other than spinal joints are named from the distal of the two bones entering into the joint; thus, a subluxation of either of the sacroiliac articulations would be spoken of as an innominate lesion, because of the two bones entering into the joint the ilium is the distal bone.

Osseous lesions are of two kinds: subluxations and traumatic lesions.

A SUBLUXATION is an immobilization of a joint in a position of normal motion, usually at the extremity of a given movement. Subluxations vary as individuals vary. One man may have an extremely flexible spine. In his case a strain would immobilize a certain articulation in a position of maximum play of the articular facets one upon the other. Another man whose spine was lacking in flexibility, a condition not always pathological but rather due to environment, occupation, hereditary tendency, would from the same amount of strain present a subluxation wherein the articulating surfaces were immobilized with fully one-half of their faces in apposition. In short, lesion means immobilization and there can be no mathematically exact limit placed upon the changes that will be found in any joint the result of a given offensive force.

A TRAUMATIC LESION is one in which the articulating surfaces of the joint are immobilized in a position physiologically abnormal to the joint and is always the result of force applied in a direction ordinarily impossible to the planes and axes of the joint. There are usually two kinds of traumatic lesions:

1. Rotation traumatic lesions, occurring in the
    a. Lumbar area, produced by forced rotation with the patient in the flexed or erect position.
    b. Lower thoracic area, produced by forced rotation with the patient in the position of flexion.

2. Sidebending traumatic lesions, occurring in the thoracic area above the eighth thoracic vertebra, produced by forced side-bending with the patient in the erect or hyperextended position.

Osseous lesions are acute or chronic according to whether or not they are of recent production, or whether or not there has been a pathological defensive reaction in the surrounding tissues. In acute lesions the effects are those which immediately follow injury and hence are inflammatory in character.

Chronic lesions are those which have been structuralized by adaptive changes in the soft tissues of the joint. To the research work of a number of osteopathists, notably among whom may be mentioned Drs. Carl P. McConnell and Frank Farmer, are we indebted for the knowledge of the conditions extant in osseous spinal lesions of the chronic type. The structural changes present are in direct ratio to the extent of the lesion for in the severe type there may be present ossification of parts of those ligaments which contain yellow elastic fibrous tissue. In the minor gradations, the following effects of lesions are characteristic: the muscle fasciculi about the joint undergo a myositis; the nerves to contractured muscles degenerate; after the muscles are dissected away from the joint, there still remains restricted articular motion; there is present much thickening of the ligaments on the side toward which the vertebra is rotated or flexed; the intervertebral discs show compression changes; the articular surfaces are not pathologically involved, synovial fluid is present, and there are no adhesions. It is unquestionably the damage done to the ligaments that maintains the osseous lesion.

THE SPINAL JOINT

Briefly, in the light of the mechanical problems it presents, it is best to review the vertebral articulation, anatomically and physiologically.

The spinal column consists of a series of bones called vertebræ, connected by fibrous and elastic structures and in larger part separated by intervertebral discs. The segmentation of the spine serves admirably the purpose for which it was made, first, to support the upper part of the body, the head, shoulder girdle, and torso; secondly, to protect the spinal cord and its membranes from injuries and concussions.

The number of vertebræ in the first years of life is thirty-three; according to their connections they have been divided into groups: seven cervical, twelve thoracic, five lumbar, five sacral, and five coccygeal. Between the fifth and tenth years, the lowest four unite to form one bone, the coccyx; between the tenth and twenty-fifth years, the five sacral unite forming a solid bone, the sacrum; the remaining twenty-four are called true vertebræ because they remain separated in the normal spine throughout life.

All the vertebræ are constructed upon the same general plan:

1. A strong body for the transmission of weight.
   a. In the lumbar area, kidney-shaped, massive, deeper in front than behind.
   b. In the thoracic area, heart-shaped, deeper behind than in front, diminishing in size gradually from the twelfth to the third.
   c. In the cervical area, small, ovoid in shape, concave transversely above, sagitally below.

2. A neural arch to cover the spinal cord, divided arbitrarily into
   a. Pedicles, containing intervertebral notches, by the opposition of which are formed intervertebral foramina for the transmission of spinal nerves and blood vessels.
   b. Laminæ.

3. Spinous and transverse processes for the attachment of muscles and ligaments; in the thoracic region the transverse processes help to support the ribs.

4. Articular processes to effect a junction of the arch with that of the vertebræ above and below, the superior articular facets facing
   a. In the cervical area backward and upward.
   b. In the thoracic area backward and outward
   c. In the lumbar area backward and inward.

The interarticular fibrocartilage or disc is an integral part of the spinal articulation. Its purpose is to give elasticity to the spinal column, to protect the spinal cord from jars, and at the same time to add strength by connecting firmly and closely every two segments. Each disc is composed of two parts, the annulus fibrosus, or annual fibrous ring, the outer layer of which is composed of dense fibrous tissue, the inner layer of fibrocartilage; the other part, the nucleus pulposus, is a pulpy substance, highly elastic, tightly compressed, so that it acts as a compression cushion upon which the bodies of the vertebræ may move. The discs are not wholly separated from the vertebræ for the reason that they are connected to the hyaline cartilage which covers, and is tightly adherent to, the surfaces of the bodies.

While the discs are shaped according to the circumference of the vertebral bodies, they are unequal in depth in the lumbar and cervical areas, being deeper in front than behind and helping in that way to form the anterior convexity of the physiological curves in those regions. In the thoracic area the discs are shallower in comparison with the bodies of the vertebræ. Of the height of the entire spine, the discs constitute one-fourth.

The ligaments of a joint have two functions, first to unite the bones entering into the joint, and secondly, to limit the movement of the joint. They are strong bands of white fibrous tissue, pliant but inextensile, and closely united to the periosteum of the bones they join. These ligaments are

1. Those connecting the bodies of the vertebræ
   a. Anterior longitudinal.
   b. Posterior longitudinal.
   c. Lateral vertebral.[1]
2. Those connecting the processes
   a. Supraspinous.
   b. Interspinous.
   c. Ligamentum nuchæ.
   d. Intertransverse.

Ligaments which fill up spaces or enter into capsules in the spinal joints are largely composed of yellow elastic tissue and are

1. Capsular.
2. Flava.

The osteopathist is much concerned with the nature of the joints of the spinal column for according to the kind of movement possible are the lesions either subluxations or traumatic lesions. The joints between the bodies of the vertebræ belong to the class

---

1. Morris's "Human Anatomy" (Jackson) 1914.

Fig. 1

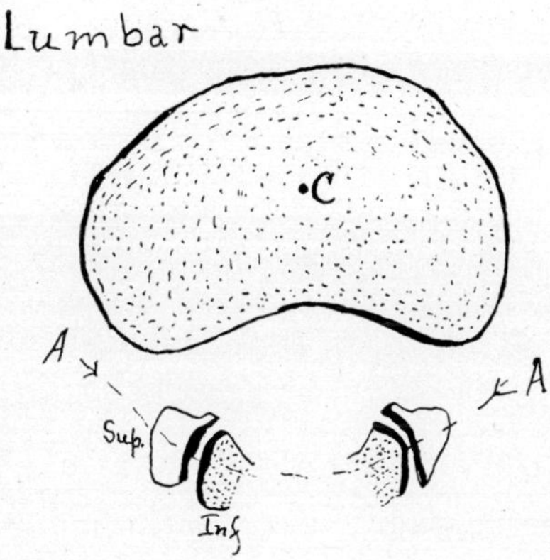

Fig. 2

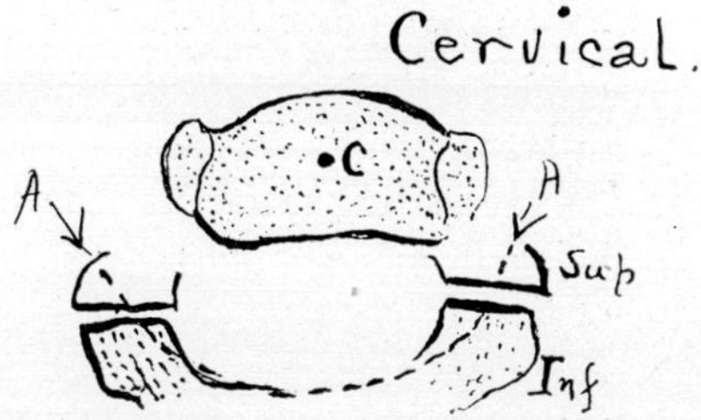

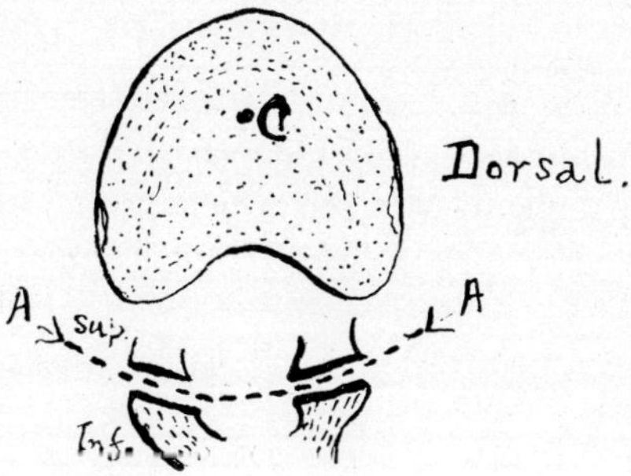

Fig. 3

Figs. 1, 2, 3.—Schematic drawings to illustrate the central point C about which the vertebra rotates. Line A-A represents the arc bisecting the planes of the articular facets in the cervical and lumbar areas and passing between the facets in the dorsal area. Sup., superior articular facets; Inf., inferior articular facets*. (After etchings in Ernest Frazer's "Anatomy of the Human Skeleton."

of amphiarthrodia,[1] joints having limited movement. The axes of motion in the spinal articulations pass through the bodies of the vertebræ, which fact assures the mechanical stability of the spinal column. It is for this purpose that discs join the bodies and where the discs are the thickest there is present the greatest amount of motion in the joints.

To the larger class of arthrodia belong the articular joints and they are characterized by a gliding of one articulating surface upon the other, the amount of movement being limited by the ligaments and the contact of osseous processes. The influence of

---

*Frazer's book is probably the best upon the osteology of man. It was published by P. Blakiston's Son & Co., 1914.

1. Anatomical descriptions in this book will be brief, with the supposition that the student undertaking the subject has spent at least one year in a thorough study of descriptive anatomy.

the articular processes upon the movements of the spinal column may be plainly seen when due consideration is given the planes[1] of the articular surfaces which limit the direction of inclination in any given movement.

It is axiomatic that the bodies of the vertebræ move least, being in and about the center of motion; the various processes of the vertebræ move more in proportion as they are farther away from the central axis, thus: in rotation in the dorsal area the spinous process of the vertebra would move in a larger arc than any line upon the posterior surface of the arch.

THE MATTER OF EQUILIBRIUM

The problem which constantly confronts man is that of maintaining the upright position, or stated in one word, balance. The difficulties under which he labors in holding himself erect may be demonstrated best by a comparison between the mechanics of the quadruped's position with that of the human.

	QUADRUPED	MAN
Spine	Horizontal	Upright
Support	Four limbs	Two limbs
Base	Large	Small
Superstructure	Low	High
Mass supported	Moderate	Large
Thorax	Swung between supports	Disposed in line of weight
Inspiration	Ribs fall into expansion	Ribs pulled up and thorax expanded
Expiration	Ribs pulled up	Ribs fall
Viscera carried	At right angles	In long axis
Muscular effort necessary to maintain balance	Small	Great

Man's weight is disposed in a plane at right angles to that for which mechanically it was best adapted, and from the above it may thus be seen that a large number of factors enter into the matter of equilibrium and that there is required a continuous adjustment to a constantly varying position of the line of gravity.

Balance is reflex, instinctive and is maintained by means of

1. The planes of the articulating surfaces are of the utmost importance in the consideration of any articulation.

co-ordinated muscular action. Due to the segmentation of the body, there is a constant shifting of weight forces and the individual must be able to keep his center of gravity over the center of support or lose the symmetry normal to the upright position. The sum of man's experiences in maintaining equilibrium constitutes what is termed his posture, attitude, standing position.

The carriage of the body at any given period of life is resultant upon the individual's struggles with the influences of environment, occupation, diseases that weaken the organism, strains, fatigue, climatic conditions, etc. It is most noticeable in a disturbance in the curves of the spine which are directly the effect of man's effort to attain the upright position.

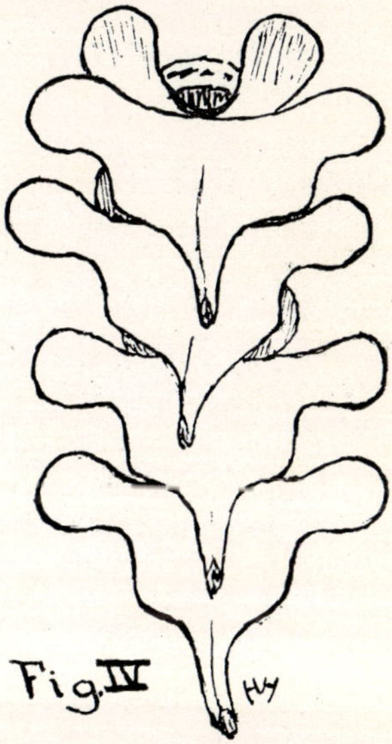

FIG. 4.—A part of the dorsal area of the spine showing a deflected spinous process of the lowest vertebra.

The normal spine has four physiological curves. Two are primary, and are so called because they appear within the first year of life, and two are secondary, the result of the child's struggle to maintain his body in the erect position. The sacral and dorsal curves are the primary ones; the cervical curve is brought about by the carriage of the head, and the lumbar curve is established after the child has learned to walk. The secondary curves are counterbalancing and may be almost wholly obliterated by placing the patient in suspension, taking the weight of his trunk off from his spine.

There is the same relation between lesions that there is between curves, primary and secondary, and the secondary lesion is always for the purpose of restoring erectness or equilibrium. A primary lesion may be defined as one that originates independently of any other lesion. A secondary lesion is one that follows a primary lesion and is compensatory or counterbalancing in character. They are further distinguished by the functional test of mobility. A primary lesion is an immobilization of a joint wherein movement is restricted or lost. A secondary lesion may show slight limitations of motion but it is not to be characterized as a lesion in the sense of complete immobilization. It may disappear in flexion or extension, in forced rotation or sidebending. At rest it appears like a primary lesion. Its diagnosis is made by palpation which is the province of the osteopathist.

OSTEOPATHIC DIAGNOSIS is the science and art of finding and defining abnormalities in organs and tissues. It embraces not alone physical diagnosis but that peculiar science originated by Andrew Taylor Still which seeks to find in spinal maladjustment a potent etiological factor in the production of disease. Osteopathy has brought to perfection the art of palpation. By it the osteopathist is able to detect the minutest deviation from the normal in structural relations and physiological action.

OSTEOPATHIC TECHNIQUE consists in definite operations for the precise adjustment of structural deviations and for the regulation of functional perversions. As a part of Osteopathic Mechanics it is concerned with the execution of definite manual procedures in exact accord with mechanical laws. To these laws has been given the term, principles of correction.

A corrective movement is one that has for its purpose the adjustment of lesion. A lesion that has been adjusted has been removed. The secondary effects, near and remote, have no further etiological foundation; but if due to habits of unbalance they persist, they may be overcome by the same principles of correction that would be applied to primary lesions.

Anatomies have established certain rules for the ready recognition of spinal areas and certain vertebræ. In his study of the spine of the living subject, the student will find them of great value.

SPINOUS PROCESS.

7th cervical .... prominent, differentiated from the 1st thoracic by the disappearance of the spine of the 6th in extension of the head.
3d dorsal .... opposite the root of the spine of the scapula.
7th dorsal......... opposite the inferior angle of the scapula.
Tip of process
  Dorsal area ..... at the level of the vertebral body next below.
  Upper dorsal .... corresponds to the head of the rib next below.

Middorsal.......corresponds with the disc between the two vertebral bodies next below its own body.
11th and 12th ...opposite the heads of the corresponding ribs.
4th lumbar......level with the highest points of the crests of the innominates.
Any lumbar ....level with the disc below the same vertebra.
Third sacral........level with the posterior superior spines of the innominates.

In osteopathic technique, the seventh cervical vertebra is regarded as a thoracic vertebra, and the twelfth thoracic as a lumbar vertebra. Each of these functionally belongs to the latter class rather than to the one of anatomical selection.

The principle of the lever is the one most commonly used in the adjustment of lesions, with that of the inclined plane, the wedge, occasionally employed. There are three classes of levers in the human body just as there are in machines, but in osteopathic mechanics the term fixed point has largely replaced the term fulcrum and in this book the extremities of the weight and power arms are designated usually as points of attack.

Standardization is the purpose of most of our recent researches in the mechanics of osteopathy but we are being constantly brought face to face with the fact that the mechanical powers of the human body vary in degree if not in kind and that the problems are yet far from being completely solved.

Bibliography: Cunningham's Anatomy, pg. 91-95; 299-309.
Deaver's Surgical Anatomy, Vol. I, pg. 412-419.
Frazer, ibid, Chap. II.
Gray's Anatomy, pg. 259-273.
Lovett's Lateral Curvature of the Spine, Chap. I.
Morris's Anatomy, pg. 31-38, 211-215, 225-232.

CHAPTER II.

THE NORMAL MOVEMENTS OF THE SPINE

The normal human spine is capable of three movements: (1) flexion; (2) extension, and (3) a compound movement, rotation-sidebending or sidebending-rotation.

FLEXION

Flexion is secured by bending the body forward, inclining the head upon the chest, the torso and pelvis upon the thighs. The back shows a marked posterior curve but the spinal column itself has less of true flexion than appears in the bent body. The amount of flexion present in any spine may be measured by a tape-line, preferably one of steel. Apply one end of the tape to the tip of any spinous process with the subject sitting in the erect position. Measure the distance between that spinous process and a certain one below. Then ask the subject to bend forward in extreme flexion and measure the distance between the same spinous processes. The difference in the two amounts will represent the extent of flexion present in that area.

The amount of flexibility in any spine differs at different periods in the life cycle. Certain occupations and diseases predispose to early rigidity. If a man is as old as his spine is rigid, by comparison we should be able to give a fairly accurate guess as to his chances for longevity.

Flexion is accomplished in the spinal joint by the gliding upward and slightly forward of the inferior articular facets upon the superior articular facets of the vertebra below. Simultaneously the intervertebral disc is compressed anteriorly and widened posteriorly, becoming wedge-shaped with the base of the wedge posterior. The posterior ligaments of the articulation are stretched. Due to the consistency of the disc and to the pull of muscles producing flexion,[1] the anterior inferior margin of the

1. Flexion of the spine is produced by the action of the following muscles: sterno-cleido-mastoid, rectus capitis anticus major, longus colli et capitis, scaleni, psoas magnus, psoas parvus, and the abdominal muscles.

body of the upper vertebra projects slightly anterior to the anterior superior margin of the vertebra below so that as a unit the vertebra may be said to have moved slightly forward.

By reason of the approximation of the bodies of the vertebræ to which it is attached, the anterior longitudinal ligament becomes somewhat relaxed and should the articulation become immobilized in this position, adaptive shortening and thickening would result.

It is a matter of muscular and ligamentous tone how much movement takes place between the articular facets of any spinal joint. Experience confirms the opinion that the movement is complete when the lower one-third of the inferior articular facet remains in apposition with the upper one-third of the corresponding superior facet. Much less than this amount is common to the average spine.

In the cervical and lumbar areas flexion is free; in the thoracic area of the spine flexion is restricted, due to the attachment of the ribs; especially is this true of the upper six thoracic articulations.

Flexion subluxations are common to the lumbar and thoracic areas but infrequent in the cervical region for the reason that blows to the skull or other strains are more likely to cause lesions of the occipitoatloid or cervicodorsal articulations.

EXTENSION

Extension is a backward bending of the spinal column and is a restricted movement throughout the entire spine, due to (1) the interference of bony processes, and (2) to the tenacity of the anterior longitudinal ligament. It is the least common of the movements of the spine beyond the action of making erect the spinal column after flexion. The spinal articulations are rarely carried beyond the normal apposition of articulating surfaces, that apposition which is present when man sits or stands erect. The amount of extension in any area may be determined by measurement with the tape.

Extension[1] is accomplished in the spinal articulation by a

1. Extension in the spinal column is the result of the action of the following muscles: splenius capitis et cervicis, spinalis, sacrospinalis, semispinalis capitis, cervicis, et dorsi, multifidus, rotatores, levatores costarum, intertransversarii, and quadratus lumborum.

gliding backward of the inferior articular facets upon the superior articular facets of the vertebra below and is a movement of very slight extent. Simultaneously the intervertebral disc is compressed posteriorly and stretched anteriorly, so that it becomes slightly wedge-shaped with the base of the wedge anterior. The anterior longitudinal and the lateral vertebral ligaments are stretched and the posterior ligaments relaxed. Should immobilization in this position occur, the posterior group of ligaments would in time become shortened and thickened. The inferior anterior margin of the body of the vertebra does recede slightly from the anterior superior margin of the vertebra below, so that the vertebra as a unit is actually slightly posterior to the vertebra below.

Extension is free in the cervical and lumbar areas, but restricted in the dorsal area. Extension subluxations are found in the thoracic and lumbar areas; very rarely in the cervical region.

ROTATION

Rotation,[1] it has been stated, is always one part of a compound movement, the other part being sidebending. The reason for the union of these two movements is found in the mechanism of the spinal column as a whole. The spine is not composed of a series of rectangular cubes disposed in parallel lines upon a central axis of rotation. It is rather a series of wedges, bony and cartilaginous, united quite firmly together by tenacious bands which help to maintain these wedges in physiological curves, which have been determined by the shape of the component parts and preserved in the living body by the integrity of muscles and ligaments. They act together as a flexible rod, which being bent in one plane cannot be turned in another without twisting. The constant expression of this torsion is secondary sidebending when rotation is the initiative movement, and is secondary rotation when sidebending is the initiative movement.

The human spine responds to rotation differently in different areas depending upon the plane of the articulating surfaces and

1. For detailed description see Robert W. Lovett's "Lateral Curvature of the Spine," 2nd edit., page 29.

upon the position of the spine, whether erect, flexed, or hyper-extended.

EXPERIMENT I.—Ask the subject, whose back should be well exposed, to sit upon a stool and hold the spine comfortably erect. He may place his hands upon his head, elbows forward, to spread

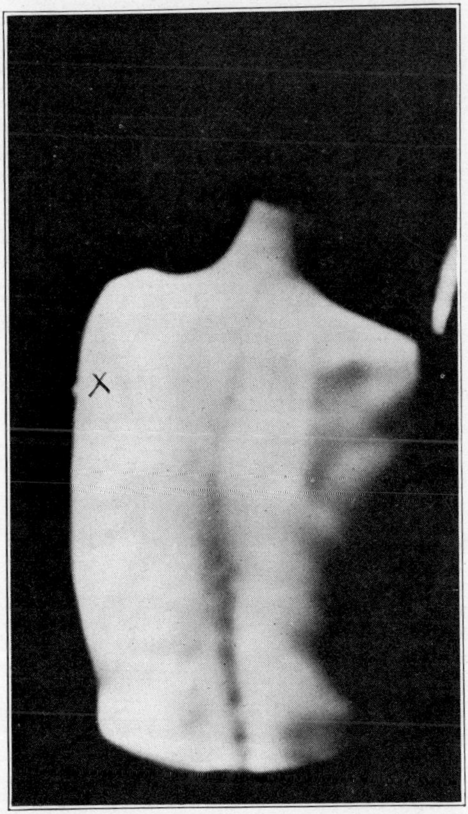

FIG. 5.—The artificial production of a rotation curvature. The hand of the demonstrator who is turning the subject to the right is indicated by the cross. This illustrates experiment I.

the scapulæ. Direct the subject to turn his head and torso to the right and ask him to hold the position. A curvature will be seen in the thoracic area, from the first to the tenth vertebræ inclusive, with the convexity of the curve to the left, the concavity to the right. Further examination shows a prominence of the ribs upon the right and a flattening of the ribs upon the left. To determine this, it may be necessary to stand above the patient and look down upon his back, making a comparison between the two sides. The greatest deviation from the normal will be found at the apex of the curve. Dr. Lovett and others have designated the side of the prominent ribs as the high side,[1] in contradistinction to the flattening that has taken place upon the other side.

This experiment demonstrates that the bodies of the thoracic vertebræ have turned toward the right, the concavity of the curve;

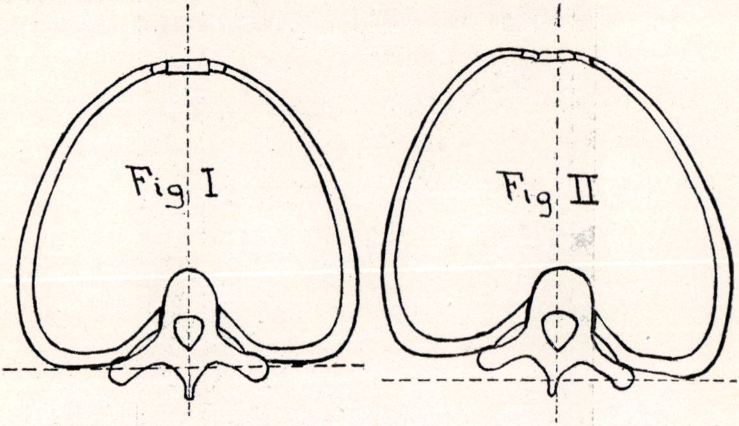

FIG. 6.—The ribs of a person facing forward are indicated in Fig. I. The person who rotates his trunk to the right turns the vertebræ and ribs as indicated by Fig. II.

the spinous processes have turned in a reverse direction; in turning, the right transverse processes were compelled to move backward, the left ones forward; the ribs articulating with the right transverse processes were pulled backward, and those upon the left side were pushed forward by the rotation forward of the transverse processes on that side.

Further, if the bodies of the vertebræ rotated to the concavity of the curve, and that concavity was upon the right, then the right transverse processes must have approached one another; the converse is true,—if the left transverse processes, the side of the convexity, took part in the general sidetilting of the vertebræ, then they must have been separated and are further apart, one

1. The term high side has been so universally adopted and is so well understood that it will not be placed in quotation marks in this book.

from another. The corresponding ribs would also manifest the same changes.

Experiment II.—Let the demonstrator stand to the right side of the subject and grasping him by the shoulders, forcibly rotate him further to the right. It will be observed that rotation may thus be made to take place in the lumbar area.

In a subject with a flexible spine, forcible rotation would be without danger, but in those whose spines were more or less rigid, it would be possible to produce traumatic rotation lesions among the lumbar articulations.

The lumbar area, with the subject in the erect position, is locked against rotation.

Experiment III.—With the subject seated, direct him to bend forward in moderate flexion and then to rotate the trunk as before. The area that responds to rotation is less in extent than in the erect position. Greater flexion still further restricts it, until in the position of extreme forward flexion, it is doubtful if rotation exists lower than the third thoracic. The high side is upon the concavity, showing that the vertebral bodies have rotated to the concavity.

By forward flexion, the lower thoracic and lumbar areas are locked against rotation.

Experiment IV.—Place straps across the subject's thighs, attached to rings in the floor, so that his pelvis may be fixed and he shall have no sensation of unbalance in any position. Ask the subject to carry his torso back in extension. Direct him to turn his body to the right. It may be plainly seen that the torso as a whole has rotated upon an axis at the dorsolumbar junction. In the average subject rotation in hyperextension takes place between the eleventh thoracic and the second lumbar only. The same signs are present as in rotation in the erect position. The high side in the lumbar area is produced by the pushing backward of the muscle mass by the transverse processes.

Forcible rotation with a patient in this position might produce a traumatic lesion among the lower lumbar articulations.

By hyperextension the upper and middorsal and the lower lumbar areas are locked against rotation.

Rotation in the cervical area is largely a matter of the atlanto-axial articulation, but may be effected among the cervical joints and is present in the occipitoatloid articulation in extreme rotation of the head. We shall consider here rotation as it occurs in the cervical area.

EXPERIMENT V.—With the subject sitting, the demonstrator stands behind him and places both thumbs, one over the other, upon a cervical spinous process, preferably the sixth cervical. He then pushes aside the sternocleidomastoid muscles and places the radial side of the index fingers against the anterior tubercles of the transverse processes from the axis to the sixth cervical. It is easier for some demonstrators to place the cushions of the finger tips upon the same bony processes, to which no objection can be made if the pressure exerted is exceedingly light. Palpation is more successful the lighter the application of force, a fact often ignored by students.

Ask the subject to turn his face slowly to the right. Immediately it is to be noticed that the distance between the thumb and the fingers of the left hand, antero-posteriorly, is greater than that between the thumb and fingers of the right hand; that while there has been an increase upon the left there has been no appreciable change in the distance upon the right. Ask the subject to turn the face again to the front and repeat the experiment. Note subsequently that the vertical height upon the left has increased, upon the right there is apparently a slight decrease and careful palpation may explain the fact since a curvature may now be detected in the cervical region with the concavity upon the right, the convexity upon the left.

Ask the subject to flex the head forward and attempt rotation, whereupon it will be found that flexion limits cervical rotation. Ask him to hyperextend the head, and again, hyperextension will be found to limit rotation, though not as perceptibly as flexion limits it.

By the increase of depth antero-posteriorly upon the left, it has been demonstrated that the left transverse processes have moved forward, which in turn signifies that the bodies have rotated toward the right, the side of the concavity of the curve. The unchanged condition of depth upon the right demonstrates that the axis of motion for cervical rotation is a vertical one passing through the articular facets upon that side. The presence of convexity upon the left and concavity upon the right demonstrates that secondary sidebending has taken place. The increased height vertically upon the left, together with the increased depth antero-posteriorly upon the same side, demonstrates that each inferior articular facet upon the left has moved upward and forward upon the corresponding superior articular facet of the vertebra below.

We may summarize our conclusions:

I. In rotation-sidebending, the bodies of the vertebræ rotate to the concavity of the curve.

II. The high side is upon the concavity.

III. Each vertebra as a whole has tilted and rotated toward the right.

a. The right transverse process has moved backward and has approached the one below.

b. The left transverse process has moved forward and has separated from the one below.

IV. Flexion lessens rotation from below upward.

V. Hyperextension lessens rotation in the cervical area and in the dorsal and lumbar areas restricts rotation to the dorso-lumbar junction only.

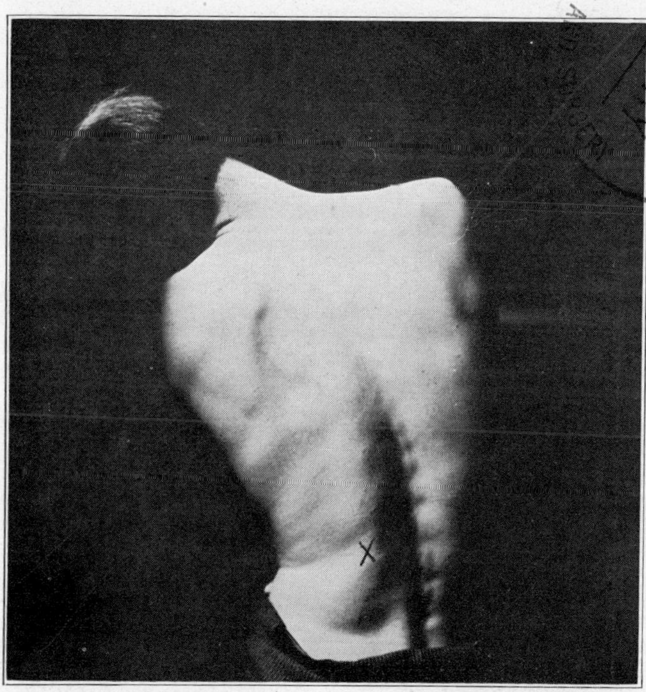

Fig. 7.—This represents the concave torsion in the lumbar area in sidebending in the erect position. The cross is placed upon the high side. This illustrates experiment VI.

SIDEBENDING

Initiative sidebending[1] is accompanied by secondary rotation. It is, therefore, not a simple movement of the spine but part of a compound movement. In other texts, it has been spoken of as lateral flexion, or as abduction.

EXPERIMENT VI.—Ask the subject seated upon the stool, with pelvis fixed by straps across the thighs fastened to rings in the floor, to bend sidewise to the right. For the purpose of exact observation, add support beneath the right shoulder so that the subject shall expend no muscular effort to prevent falling. This is particularly essential since the foreign orthopedists have failed to draw tenable conclusions in regard to the conduct of the vertebræ in sidebending. The human spine behaves much better in experimentation when freed from undue muscular action.

A curvature is seen in the lumbar area of the spine, including the last two or three thoracic spinous processes, concave to the right, with the high side upon the concavity of the curve. Figure 7 represents what is seen in this experiment. Spinal columns having more rigidity will react less completely to sidebending in this position.

EXPERIMENT VII.—With the subject and demonstrator as in experiment V, ask the subject to bend the head to the right, increased vertical height among the transverse processes and the convexity of a curve may be palpated upon the left, with no appreciable change save the formation of the concavity of a curve on the right. Ask the subject to raise the head and repeat the sidebending. Palpating for change in the depth antero-posteriorly, it may be noted that there is present some increase upon the left but no appreciable change upon the right. The results of this experiment are so constant in respect to the signs with that obtained in the study of rotation, that we may adopt the same conclusions.

EXPERIMENT VIII.—With the patient seated as in experiment VI, ask him to hyperextend the spine and then bend laterally. A curvature is seen in the lower lumbar area and the high side is on the concavity of the curve.

Hyperextension limits sidebending to the lumbar area and the thoracic area by hyperextension is locked against sidebending.

EXPERIMENT IX.—With the subject seated, ask him to bend forward in moderate flexion and then to sidebend his torso to the right. A curvature appears convex to the left, concave to the right, in extent from the first to the eighth or tenth thoracic. The high side is upon the left.

1. See Lovett, ibid, p. 25.

Since the high side means that side toward which the bodies of the vertebræ have rotated, it is to be remarked in this instance that the bodies of the vertebræ have rotated to the convexity of the curve. The left transverse processes have moved backward, the right transverse processes have moved slightly forward; while the spinous processes form the convexity of the curve upon the left, each by the turning of the vertebral body has turned in a reverse direction toward the right, a point to be remembered in the consideration of the subluxation of a single vertebra in flexed sidebending-rotation.

Each vertebra taking part in the sidebending has sidetilted to the right but is rotated toward the left. Due to its position, the right transverse processes approach one another, the left transverse processes are separated. The intervertebral disc between any two of the vertebræ is compressed upon the right, stretched upon the left.

The reason for the rotation to the left is due to the fact that in flexion the bodies of the vertebræ have by the compression of the discs anteriorly been brought together. Sidebending adds compression upon the discs on the right and the bodies of the vertebræ responding to the combination of forces move in the path of least resistance, the convexity of the curve.

We may summarize our conclusions:

I. Sidebending-rotation in the erect position occurs in the dorsolumbar and cervical areas only.

II. The bodies of the vertebræ rotate to the side of the concavity.

III. Flexion lessens sidebending in extent to the upper and middorsal areas, and the bodies of the vertebræ rotate to the side of the convexity.

- a. Each vertebra as a whole has tilted toward the right and rotated toward the left.
    1. The right transverse process is approximated to the one below.
    2. The left transverse process is prominent and separated from the one below.

IV. Hyperextension lessens sidebending in extent, confines it to the lumbar area of the spine, and the bodies of the vertebræ rotate to the concavity of the curve. The twelfth dorsal acts as a lumbar vertebra, a fact that has been noted before.

CHAPTER III.

LATERAL CURVATURE OF THE SPINE

Lateral curvature[1] of the spine is a condition in which there is a lateral deviation with torsion of a series of vertebral bodies from the mesial plane of the body. The spinous processes appear as a curved line in the back. The curvature is constant in the erect position and is distinguished as functional or postural when it disappears in recumbency and as structural when it is permanent in whatsoever position the body may be placed.

Curvature was recognized by the ancients, who gave much consideration to the causal factors and the mechanical problems in correction. Hippocrates in the fourth century B. C. was probably the first writer to describe curvature of the spine. With him originated the term scoliosis, from a Greek word meaning to twist or bend. He gave as his opinion that the first cause of scoliosis was a dislocation of a vertebra. This was the accepted idea for many centuries. Ambroise Pare, in the first half of the sixteenth century, not only presented many arguments in favor of this theory but also claimed a spinal subluxation origin for most diseases. In 1641, Riolan, in France, advanced as causal factors, the wearing of clothing with improper constrictions and the excessive use of the right arm. Glisson in 1660 suggested rickets as an additional cause. Andre, the man who gave to the world the word, "orthopedic,"[2] writing in 1741, ascribed curva-

---

1. Bibliography.—Lateral Curvature of the Spine, R. W. Lovett, second edition, 1912. P. Blakiston's Son & Co., Philadelphia.

Scoliosis, George M. Laughlin. 1914. American School of Osteopathy, Kirksville, Mo.

Orthopedic Surgery, Royal Whitman, 1910. Lea & Febiger, Philadelphia.

Surgery, Principles and Practice, A. P. C. Ashhurst. 1914. Lea & Febiger, Philadelphia.

The American Journal of Orthopedic Surgery, July, 1913. P. Blakiston's Son & Co., Philadelphia.

Lateral Curvature of the Spine and Flat-Foot, J. S. K. Smith, 1911. Wm. Wood & Co., New York.

2. "L'Orthopedie est l'art de prevenir et de corriger dans les enfants les deformities du corps." The word comes from two Greek words meaning "straight" and "child".

ture to the use of high heels, bad sitting postures, and the irritation of hemorrhoids. In 1779, Percival Pott, an English physician, eliminated caries of the spine from the general classification of scoliosis, and on account of his researches into that condition, left a memory of his work in the common name for tuberculosis of the spine, Pott's disease. Wullstein, a decade ago, added much to the understanding of the mechanics underlying the production of curvature by his experiments with the spines of young dogs. Boehm in 1906 by separating the etiology of scoliosis into congenital and acquired classes, called attention to malformations of bone as a primary cause.

FUNCTIONAL CURVATURE

The line of gravity which represents the concentration of the weight forces acting upon the body, is constantly shifting because the body is a segmented structure. Man must be able to adjust the segments one to another momentarily to maintain his equilibrium. This action is reflex, instinctive, and depends upon his having a normal body and an intact nervous system. Let disturbance in either take place and curvature is an early effect. Its mechanism follows definite laws and may be demonstrated by a study of functional curvatures experimentally produced and by inductive reasoning and an examination of patients presenting the structual type of curvature.

In the study of the normal movements of the spine, we have seen that in the erect position either rotation or sidebending, when held immobilized for the purpose of observation, presents a curve in the spine with the constant sign of the high side on the concavity.

Careful examination of a patient with the functional type of curvature will reveal that such a case presents the same picture so that we may conclude that as a result of partial immobilization the vertebræ remain twisted in curvature and that the production has been in accord with the mechanical laws governing the movements of the spine, sidebending in the lumbar area, rotation in the dorsal area. The question to be answered is what may be the force or cause resulting in immobilization.

EXPERIMENT I.—Place upon the floor a brick or block of wood three or four inches in height. Ask the subject to stand, with his weight equally divided, with the right foot upon the block, the left foot upon the floor at a distance of eighteen inches away from the block. A curvature in the dorsolumbar area is produced, with the concavity to the right. The high side is upon the concavity, showing that the vertebral bodies have rotated to that side. The right hip is noticeably prominent, the waist-line apparently deeper, while upon the left side the hip is less prominent, the waist-line seemingly shallower. We have here the counterpart of a patient with a postural curvature in the same area.

By this experiment it has been demonstrated that one of the causes may be a lengthening of one of the supporting sides, or the same effect could be produced by shortening the other side.

Any one of the following causes would operate in the same way: sacroiliac lesion; flat-foot; stiff knee or ankle from arthritis, tuberculosis, or other infective process; contraction of muscles from pain, as in sciatica or in abscess formation; fracture; dislocation; alteration in soft tissues as in cicatrix or growth; muscular atrophy or spasticity from paralysis; difference in the length of the bones of the leg, or congenital malformations.

Faulty habits enter largely into the production of curvature. There are postures in standing, sitting, and lying which if maintained for any considerable length of time, cause adaptive muscular shortening upon one side, with the formation of a concavity laterally in the spinal column. Some of these habits are the result of carelessness, some are due to fatigue, mental or physical; some to weakness from diseases which lower the general vitality of the body as malnutrition, rachitis, lack of oxygenation, and digestive ailments; some to occupations requiring the individual to hold a part of his body in a position of strain for hours at a time; some to errors of refraction or disturbance in hearing in one ear. School furniture may be a cause in not suiting the size of the child who sits for hours in the classroom. Blackboards having upon them a lesson to be copied may be placed at one side instead of in front of the child.

Of the habits which result in postural curvature of the dorsolumbar area may be mentioned standing with the weight upon one foot, sitting on the foot, or with a knee crossed over the other, sleeping upon the side with the head high or with the shoulder lifted by a pillow. These are common faults in adults and hence nearly all those who develop the dorsolumbar lateral curvature after the age of twenty do so from one of these causes.

Children err in attitudes from shyness, restlessness, or weakness. They react to uncomfortable clothing by a twist or a bend. Tight clothing across the chest prevents the normal development of the spinal musculature. A tight armhole will cause a child to carry the shoulder high. Straps too far out upon the shoulders where weight should not be placed during the years of growth, cause a sagging of the shoulders and indirectly a dropping of one more than the other. An ill-fitting shoe may be the first cause of inequality of support from the base. Children are clever imitators, unconsciously to a great extent. They easily fall into the faulty postures of their parents or teachers.

Not all faults in habit lead to lateral curvatures for accompanying growth there is usually development of strength and in athletic sports and games, action is demanded of all muscles with the result that the lagging one reacts strongly to stimuli and in time equilibrium is restored.

Dorsolumbar lateral curves may be due to horseback-riding with a side-saddle. Sitting at ease in a slumped position against the arm of a chair while reading or sewing is a frequent source of postural curvature in middle-aged women. The congenital anomaly of a lumbar rib is a cause of unbalance in that region of the spine with subsequent lateral curvature.

Weight is the primary factor in the production of all curvatures. Experiments have been made with cadavers upon whose shoulders have been placed heavy loads, usually of eighty pounds. A bending forward of the dorsal area, an increased lordosis in the lumbar region, were immediate results, followed by lateral bending or rotation. Ever so slight an increase in the weight on one or the other side brings out a lateral curvature.

The carrying of the head, shoulder girdle, and thorax does not seem much in itself, but in the presence of weakness, the load is greater than the muscles' strength can bear. It may be stated as a corollary that the spine is only as strong as its weakest muscle. It follows that any disturbance in the musculature would cause an immediate disturbance in the spinal articulations controlled by that muscle. Antagonistic action of flexors and extensors maintains the spine erect. Antagonistic action of the muscles of the two sides of the spine prevents lateral bending. Let one muscle in any group be paralyzed or injured to the extent of lost tone and unbalance will result. Curvature is the gross effect of disturbed equilibrium.

Sometimes at birth certain muscles have been found paralyzed and that individual necessarily grows up with unavoidable curvature, usually structural in type. In the same way later paralysis, anterior poliomyelitis, when it manifests paralysis of the spinal muscles, causes a lateral curvature. Any irritation located in the back or lateral thoracic wall will cause an inequality in the action of the spinal muscles and thoracic curvature will result. Among such causes may be found lesions or fractures of the ribs; empyema usually followed by a resection of a rib; pleuritic inflammations, abscesses, or adhesions; wounds; scars; intercostal neuraliga; appendicitis; ovarian and uterine diseases causing pain upon one side, and disease of a kidney.

Curvatures in the upper thoracic or cervical areas are not as common as those below. Any inequality in the weight of the head or interference with the carriage of the shoulder girdle predisposes to changed relations among the vertebræ. The causes recognized by osteopathic physicians are lateral occipital lesions, lateral atlas lesions, anterior cervical lesions, torticollis, injuries to the shoulder joint causing pain and disturbance in mobility, inflammations in the head as mastoiditis or of the lateral chain of cervical lymphatics. A cervical rib, a congènital anomaly, almost always causes an irritation which leads, by the individual's effort in securing relief in a changed position or carriage, to curvature at the cervicothoracic junction.

From the causes above given no definite time can be stated as that wherein there would be the complete development of either the functional or structural type of curvature. Rapidity of change from the normal is marked in the frail child, the anemic girl, the lazy man or woman who has faulty habits of posture. Environment, nutrition, fresh air, systematic exercise, all are factors in delaying the progress of any case. Except in a few cities where compulsory examination of the spines of school children is required, curvatures are not discovered early but rather at the beginning of adolescence when a dressmarker or a tailor remarks upon the presence of a high hip or low shoulder. It is not usually then that a spinal examination is made. Later, only when by reason of the remark of some friend or relative that there seems to be some distortion in the patient's body, does the patient seek advice. As the treatment for the two types of curvatures is entirely unlike, a careful examination must be made and the diagnosis be established without doubt.

Functional curvature may be defined as a partial immobilization of a part of the spine in a position of physiological lateral bending or rotation. It occurs in all areas of the spine and is named according to the convexity of the curve and the area wherein it appears. A right cervical curve means a curve convex to the right in the cervical area of the spine as seen from behind the patient. Others are named accordingly:

Right cervicodorsal: convexity to the right, curve among the lower cervical and upper dorsal vertebræ.

Right dorsal: convexity to the right, curve among the dorsal vertebræ.

Right dorsolumbar: convexity to the right, curve among the lower dorsal and upper lumbar vertebræ.

Right lumbar: convexity to the right, curve in the lumbar area.

A long postural, total, or functional curvature is one involving practically all of the lumbar and dorsal areas, in extent usually from the upper or middorsal region to the lumbosacral joint. It is one that is common among women between the ages of twenty and forty as the result of a faulty habit in standing or sitting. The patients are otherwise quite healthy.

The characteristics of a left total curve are as follows:

1. A curve of the dorsal and lumbar areas with the convexity to the left.

2. The high side is on the right.

3. The left shoulder is elevated.

4. The right side of the shoulder girdle has been carried backward and the left side forward.

5. Lateral flexion to the right is freer than lateral flexion to the left.

6. The curvature disappears upon recumbency.

In a case of long standing, as in the class of patients of the age of forty, sometimes the curvature does not entirely disappear upon assuming the prone position, which is a manifestation of the strength of the contractures of the muscles on the side of the concavity.

When a total curve appears in a child or adolescent, it does not always remain of that type. That which usually happens is a transition to the double or figure-S curve, occasionally to the triple curve. The second curve is due to the subconscious efforts of the patient to square his shoulder girdle with his pelvis. It is plain from the above description of a patient with a total curvature that, in order to face forward in standing or walking, he must either twist his pelvis and legs, or otherwise he must face to the right slightly at all times when in the erect position. Without conscious effort he turns that portion which is more easily moved, the shoulder girdle. In so doing he elevates the right shoulder and rotates it to the front, he depresses the left shoulder and turns it backward, and he rotates the bodies of the vertebræ from the right to the left, producing by the law of rotation a curve, concave to the left, with the high side upon the concavity. There are then present two curves in the spine, one to the left in the dorsolumbar area, and one to the right in the upper dorsal area and sometimes including the cervicodorsal area.

EXPERIMENT II.—With the subject standing with one foot upon the block and the other on the floor, as in experiment I, after the spine has settled into a left dorsolumbar or total curvature, ask the subject to square his shoulders with his pelvis by turning the shoulder girdle to the left. It may be necessary for him to fold his arms across his chest or clasp his hands behind his neck in order to expose the interscapular area for observation. A curve will be found in the dorsal area, of less extent than the one below and having all the characteristics of a physiological, simple dorsal curve.

In the patient with a like condition the curves are much more easily detected for the reason that there have been muscular shortenings which preserve the changed relations whenever the spine is held in the erect position. In many of these patients, with a Webster record,[1] a little of the double curve remains when the patient assumes the prone position. This shows that the muscular contractions on the concavities are very strong.

Double curves are named according to the convexity and the area; a right lumbar left dorsal curve would be interpreted to mean a curvature in the lumbar area with the convexity to the right and a curvature in the dorsal area with the convexity to the left. Triple curves are designated in the same way, are less frequent than the double curves, and usually involve the lower cervical area or the cervicodorsal junction in the uppermost of the three curves.

EXPERIMENT III.—Repeat experiment II. At its conclusion ask the subject to bend forward in moderate flexion. The curve remains and the rotation of the bodies does not change.

By the maintenance of inequality in base, there is the same amount of pull on the vertebræ that there would be in a functional curve of long standing with the muscles on the concavity contractured.

EXAMINATION OF A PATIENT WITH CURVATURE

The usual age of the patient brought to a physician for treatment for curvature is from five to twenty-one. In this country the larger number of these patients are females but abroad where military service is demanded of all healthy males, the percentage is stated to be twenty-four males to every seventeen females.

The patient should have the entire back bared with only a thin covering over the chest so that each dorsal segment may be examined in detail. For females a short skirt gathered into an elastic band at the waist is the best apparel. For males short trousers are to be preferred, for examination of the feet in the standing position is an essential.

1. Dr. C. G. Webster of Carthage, N. Y., has devised an excellent method of preserving records of the spines of the patients he examines. The patient is placed prone upon a flat table, with the head hanging over at one end. A wide strip of adhesive tape is applied to the spine. Markings about the spinous processes are then made with an indelible pencil which has not too sharp a point. The plumb-line is then used to sketch the normal sagital line of the trunk. The tape is removed and deviations verified by osteopathic palpation of the vertebral processes.

The physical condition should be first taken into account, nutrition, size, development according to statistics for age, color, respiratory capacity, condition of the heart, pulse, vision in each eye, hearing of each ear, general carriage of the body, condition of the arches of the feet, comparison of the length of the legs,[1] manner of dress with especial attention to the way the underclothing and hosiery are supported. The nervous condition of the patient may be arrived at after the manner of the average tests applied in the examination of such patients.

While the case history is being recited, observation should be made of the patient who is asked to sit at ease. If he has faulty posture in sitting, it will be manifest after the first embarrassment wears off. Ask him to walk across the room and stand with his back toward the physician. Two or three minutes later relaxation will take place and he will manifest those signs which brought him for examination. Then should follow the determination of the actual condition.

Standing in front, the physician notes—

A. Lack of symmetry in the general outline of the body.
   1. The trunk shows a lateral displacement.
   2. One shoulder may be higher.
   3. One hip is more prominent.

Standing behind the patient it may be noted that—

B. A curvature exists in the spine.
   1. Area of involvement.
   2. The presence of a high side
      a. Upon the concavity.
      b. Upon the convexity.

C. The position of the scapulæ and their relative distance from the spine.

D. The position of the head, whether held in rotation or sidebending.

Standing above the patient and looking down upon his back, one should note—

E. The relation of the shoulder girdle to the pelvic girdle, whether one is square with the other, or whether one shoulder has rotated forward, the other backward.

1. The length of the legs may be fairly correctly measured by placing one end of a steel tape-line at the anterior superior spine of the ilium and noting the distance to the internal malleolus of the leg of the same side. The usual method of comparing the length by measuring the heels together is inexact and unreliable.

A perpendicular or plumb-line should then be erected from the cleft between the buttocks and held by one end at a point representing the top of the spinal column. A line may be traced down the middle of the back with a dermatographic pencil for the estimation of the deviation of the apex of each curve from the median line of the back. If the patient has a double curve, the extent of each curve should be noted and a record of all the findings made.

The patient should then be asked to bend forward in flexion and again the physician should note—

F. The permanency of the curve,
   1. It disappears.
   2. It is materially lessened.
   3. It does not change.

G. The patient stands with his feet apart, bends forward and the same notations are made regarding the permanency of the curve.

H. The Sayre head-sling is applied, weight is taken off from the spine, and the same notations are made.

I. The patient is asked to lie prone upon the table and again its permanency or lack of permanency is noted.

Records may be made by photograph or by X-radiance, in each case with the patient sitting with support applied laterally to the thorax so that the position may be held with ease and without wavering. A modification of the Webster record has been used by the author for keeping permanent records of the spines of these patients. The adhesive tape is applied with the patient seated, with his chest and forehead supported by photographer's rests, with the arms crossed in the lap. As the case responds to treatment, other records may be made and will serve as tests of complete correction. These are of value chiefly in making records of the functional type of curvature.

The differential diagnosis of a functional curvature is established by the presence of the following signs:

1. The high side upon the concavity of the curve.
2. Complete disappearance of curvature in the prone position.

TREATMENT

The osteopathic treatment of functional curvature is manifestly more successful than that of any other school of therapeutics for the reason that with the basic understanding which every physician of the osteopathic school has of the mechanics of the human body, he best knows how to remove the cause, how to correct the deviation of anatomical parts by the scientific application of mechanical laws, and, following the re-establishment of normal relations, how to advise against a return of the former condition.

To remove the cause is the first essential and treatment for such a purpose is to be classified as adjustive, surgical, or postural, according to what the cause is. Lesions must be adjusted, growths and congenital anomalies removed, tendons transplanted whenever possible for the sake of changing paralyzed conditions, defective eyesight or hearing given attention, inequalities of base overcome by lifts in the shoes, raised heels, or the adjustment of a flat arch. In the changing of habits of attitude, the physician must secure the cooperation of the patient for without it little can be accomplished that is permanent. Patients should be impressed with the importance of overcoming these faults and also be warned that any return to them will result in a recurrence of the curvature.

If the condition of health in the patient is poor, the treatment must begin in a general upbuilding. In youth curvature that is not severe little affects the bodily vigor but in later life as the spinal column becomes more rigid and the intervertebral discs atrophy, the curves increase in severity and tend to induce pain in the back and discomfort from the sense of the lack of symmetry. Where the cause seems to be due to fatigue, the child must be taken out of school and given outdoor life with an entire change of environment wherever possible. The same advice may be given to the older patient.

Since weight is a large factor in producing and increasing curvature, a greater number of hours of rest in recumbency should be taken for the purpose of giving the distorted spine more rest from the weight of the head and shoulder girdle.

We may not speak of the osteopathic treatment administered to cases with functional curvature as adjustive. It is corrective in character being directed toward the reversing of the curves in accord with the laws of the normal, physiologic movements of the spine. Because of the adaptive shortening of the ligaments and the contractures of the muscles on the side of the concavity, the patient is not able to help himself by exercise alone, for it is a well-known fact that the soft tissues of the passive body are more easily stretched than those of the active individual.

The process of bringing the spine back to the normal is of necessity a gradual one. The shortening of ligaments and muscles has been mentioned and offers one of the first problems in treatment. The author does not favor massage but in its stead recommends stretching of muscle fasciculi and ligaments by forcible separation of origin and insertion which may be effected by putting the spine through flexion and extension and by reversing the rotation and sidebending present in the curvature. The fibrocartilages show an adaptive compression on the concavity and by the same means will be brought toward the normal.

The most important reason why the overcoming of curvature should not be forced is that the type of patient with such a condition will not warrant it. The commonest cases are those of children of all ages from the little prattling lad who is yet in a somewhat unstable equilibrium upon his feet to the high school boy or girl. These children have had an unequal chance in the game of early achievement. They have been frail else the curvature would not have appeared. The first necessity, then, in treatment is that it shall not be rough, that it shall not hurt. Children react to pain more quickly than adults, and pain, it should be remembered, prevents voluntary relaxation, produces reflex contractions, and hinders correction.

CORRECTIVE MOVEMENTS

Principles of Correction.—In the lumbar area sidebend the patient to the convexity. In the dorsal area rotate the patient to the convexity.

General Rules.—Stretch the concavity and make a new concavity on the convexity, or what in effect is the same thing, make a new convexity of the side of the concavity.

A patient, B, is assumed to have a lumbar functional curvature, convex to the left.

I. The Creeping Movement.[1]—Let B support his trunk in the horizontal position with his hands and knees on the table.

1. This corrective movement is so named because it is like in principle a valuable exercise for a patient afflicted with a lumbar curvature, convex to the left. The exercise consists in the patient's creeping in a circle with the side of the concavity outward. See Lovett, ibid, page 145, exercises XXV, XXVI, and XXVII.

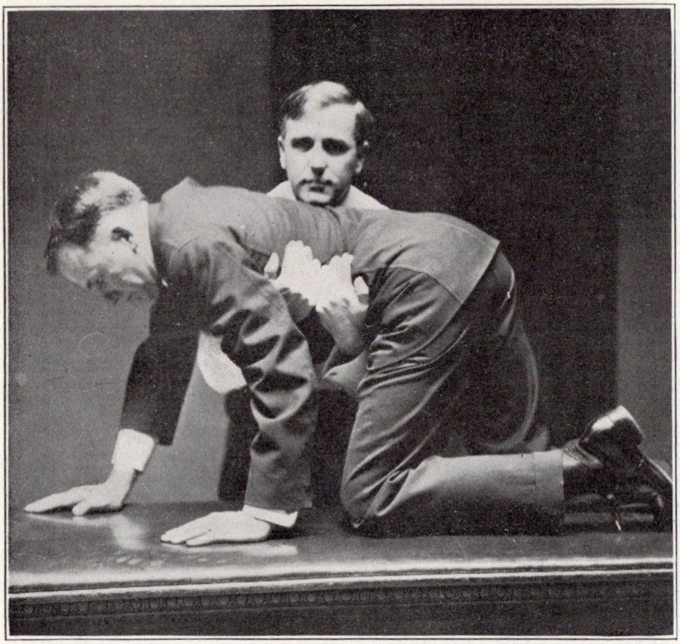

FIG. 8.—Corrective movement I for a lumbar functional curvature convex to the left.

He advances the left knee and places the left hand, palm downward, fingers pointing backward, beside it. The right knee is moved backward and the right hand is extended beyond the head with the palm downward and the fingers pointing forward. In this position the left hand and knee are close together and the right hand and knee some distance apart. The physician, O, stands at the right side of B. He places both arms under B's abdomen and grasps the side of B's thorax and waist with his hands. O's right shoulder rests in B's right axilla as a point of attack, O's left shoulder rests against the crest of B's right ilium as a second point of attack.

O pulls B towards him and at the same time he separates by strong pressure the points of attack, first, to produce a new concavity on the side of the convexity, and secondly to stretch the concavity to the fullest extent.

This corrective movement should be repeated several times

at each treatment and the patient may be advised to take the position and attempt, unaided, the movement at home between treatments.

II. HYPEREXTENSION SIDEBENDING MOVEMENT.[1]—Let the patient lie upon the table prone, with the trunk above the waist projecting over the end of the table, with the arms extended

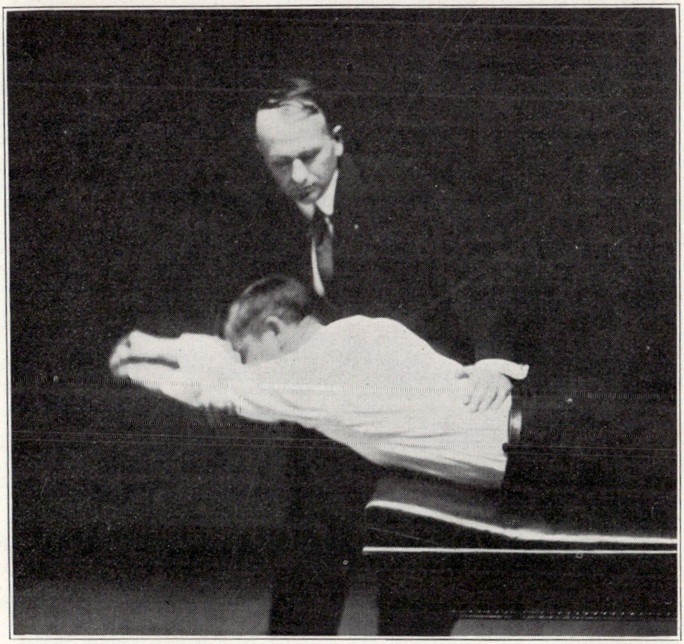

FIG. 9.—Corrective movement II, for a lumbar functional curvature convex to the right.

beyond the head and resting upon O's forearm, O standing upon the side of the convexity of the curve. O lifts B into a position of extension[2] and bends his body laterally at the waist-line toward O, while with the other hand O makes pressure against the spinous processes of the lumbar vertebræ from the side of the convexity

1. Patients relax better in some positions and in response to certain motions, therefore the student should execute with ease more than one operative movement for each condition.

2. This movement is too heavy for any but light-weight patients.

with the purpose of assisting in the attempt to make a new concavity on the side of the convexity.

Resume.—Sidebending is localized in the lumbar area by hyperextension and the dorsal area is locked by hyperextension against sidebending.

III. SIDEBENDING-ROTATION MOVEMENT.—Let the patient sit upon a stool of suitable height facing O who presses against B's knees with the purpose of fixing B's pelvis. O's right hand is placed down upon B's left shoulder, grasping the shoulder firmly as a point of attack. O's left hand passes under B's right axilla to rest upon his right shoulder blade, while B rests his right arm upon O's left arm. By pulling upward with the left hand and pushing downward with the right hand, O may bend B laterally to the left, and then slightly rotate his trunk to the same side.

Resume.—Sidebending in the lumbar area is accompanied by secondary rotation to the same side, hence as a corrective movement in the lumbar area rotation must always follow initiative sidebending.

A patient, B, is assumed to have a thoracic curvature, convex to the right.

IV. COUNTERPRESSURE MOVEMENT.—Let B sit on the end of the table. O stands to the right and slightly in front of B and passes his right arm across B's chest, under the axilla, and rests his hand upon the angles of the ribs at the apex of the thoracic curve. O places a small, firm pillow between his chest and the left anterior surface of B's thorax over the ribs diagonally in relation to the area covered by O's right hand. O reinforces his right hand with his left and exerts pressure in a straight line between the hands and the pillow gradually while B inhales with a full respiration. Let B hold his breath for a moment while O holds the pressure. As soon as O and B act synchronously, add rotation to the right at the moment of maximum pressure.

V. ROTATION RIB-LEVERAGE MOVEMENT.—Let the patient sit on the end of the table. O stands to the left of B and places his left hand upon B's right shoulder. O's right hand rests strongly upon the angles of the ribs on the high side at the apex of the curve. O rotates B's torso to the right by the pressure on the right shoulder and the left ribs.

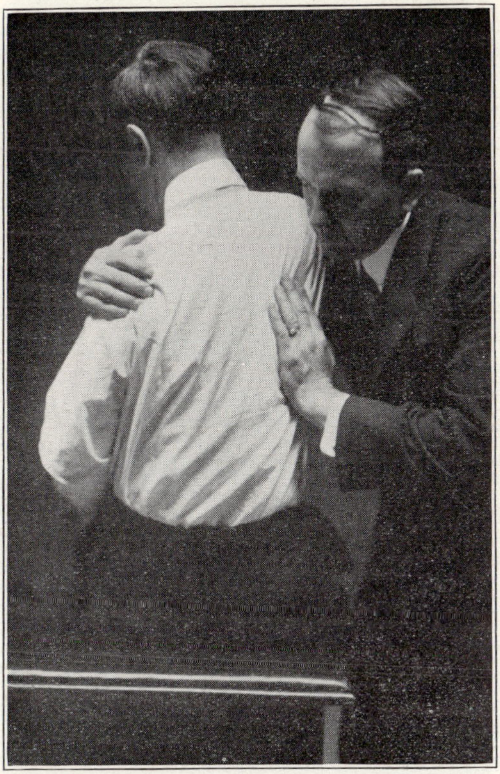

FIG. 10.—Corrective movement V for a thoracic functional curvature convex to the left.

Fig. 10 illustrates this corrective movement for a thoracic curvature the reverse of the one here described.

VI. SIMPLE ROTATION MOVEMENT.—Let the patient sit on the end of the table and cross his arms across his chest with his hands on his shoulders. O stands to the right of B grasping B's left shoulder, or stands to the right and slightly posterior to B grasping with his right hand B's left elbow. O places the thumb and thenar eminence of his left hand to the right side of the spinous processes of the vertebræ at the area of greatest de iation from the mesial line of the trunk with firm pressure against the spinous processes, while pulling on B's left shoulder or elbow, he rotates B's torso to the right.

This movement may be varied by having B reflex forward moderately before the execution of the movement if the curvature is located in the upper thoracic area but the movement must be one of pure rotation following initiative flexion.

VII. ROTATION-SIDEBENDING MOVEMENT.—Let the patient sit on the end of the table. O stands at B's right side and bends forward. B sits erect and turns slightly to rest his arms across O's back. O passes his right arm across B's chest, under his axilla, until the right hand rests over the angles of the most prominent ribs. O reaches under his left axilla with his left hand and grasps B's right wrist. O rotates B's trunk farther to the right and then sidebends him to the point of resistance.

CONCLUSION

In treatment each segment may be considered separately with the corrective movement localized for that segment. In cases in which certain articulations are less flexible than others, attention may be directed in this manner to those segments.

There is a certain kind of auxiliary treatment that is very beneficial in these cases. It consists in breathing exercises in connection with pressure against the angles of the ribs on the high side. The patient with the thoracic curve convex to the right, is asked to lie pon the face on the table. O rests his hands over the ribs on the high side and exerts five to twenty foot-pounds of pressure against the ribs at the end of B's full inspiration, and maintains the pressure while B holds his breath, relaxing the pressure at the first third of expiration. The amount of pressure to be exerted is to be determined by the age and strength of the patient. The patient may take the same exercise at home by the use of sandbags of proper weight and applied in the same place.

No treatment should be given without re-examination[1] of the patient, for there comes a time, late in the history of the case when it requires the closest scrutiny to detect that a curvature exists. This is when by treatment it has been almost entirely overcome. Therefore, it is necessary to see the spine to watch the progress of the case else at the close there would be danger of over-

1. The student should analyze again and again and at each treatment the curves his patient presents with a view to an exact understanding of the mechanics of production and correction. Repetition brings skill.

correcting, that is, causing a reverse curvature to the opposite side. In short there is no condition wherein carelessness in treatment can work greater harm. If perchance rotation or sidebending were given to the concavity, the curvature would be made worse.

Cervical curvature is usually a secondary condition, following lesions of the occipitoatloid articulation or an upper thoracic primary curvature. In any case treatment should be directed to the correction of the primary condition, after which the secondary or counterbalancing curve will take care of itself. Should it persist, however, treatment may be given in accord with the general principle of correction, rotation or sidebending in the reverse direction.

The after-treatment of functional curvature is exceedingly important for as ounces of prevention are worth more than pounds of cure, so is proper exercise and the removal of the cause vital to the permanency of the curvature correction. Atonic muscles must be stimulated to normal tone. It is not safe for some time following cure to allow the patient to enter a gymnasium for the reason that the average case requires personal attention and suitable exercises. During the latter part of the course of treatment, resistance exercises should be given for home exercise, as for example, a patient having a thoracic curvature convex to the right might strengthen the atonic muscles on the convexity by forcibly rotating the shoulders and torso to the right. A successful plan has been to have such a patient stand with back to the jamb of an open door and ask him to attempt to push the door-jamb away by turning his right shoulder backward.

Following correction, the exercises should be those of flexion, extension, and creeping in a forward direction, principally because these movements make use equally of the muscles of both halves of the trunk at the same time.

SCOLIOSIS

Of the two types of spinal malposition, functional curvature is the one which any normal spine may assume; structural curvature has no exact prototype in any position which the normal spine may take because there is always present a deformity or change in the shape of the bones. The nearest likeness to it is in the rotation of the vertebral bodies that occurs in flexion-sidebending, namely, to the convexity, but this rotation takes place without deformity.

Scoliosis, as structural curvature is preferably called, has been for convenience divided into two classes, congenital and acquired. Under the heading of congenital are those cases which may be discovered at birth or shortly afterward.

Under acquired curvature may be classified:

A. Curvatures which from weakness, bone disease, muscle atrophy, became structural without having passed through the postural stage.

B. Curvatures which at first belonged to the functional type, but later, from neglect, improper treatment, weakness of bone or soft tissues, in a short or longer process of time, became organic.

The reason for the production of congenital scoliosis is so evident as to require no elaboration, but the mechanism of change from functional to structural curvature needs demonstration.

Weakness and weight may be considered the two greatest constant factors producing deviations from the normal in the curves of the spinal column. Patients, weak from disease or fatigue, show frequently the influence of weight in the accentuation of the normal antero-posterior curves; the increased posterior thoracic curve being spoken of as a kyphosis, the increased anterior lumbar curve as a lordosis. With the addition of faulty posture, weight and fatigue bring about lateral spinal curvature. The process between this and scoliosis may be explained thus:

Constant weight bearing down upon the upper extremity of a flexible, weight-bearing arc, would cause an increase in the curve of that arc, a decrease in its radius. But when that arc is the human spine, it is not a mere line. It is composed of a series of solid bodies, held together by soft elastic tissues, rotating on an axis passing through the anterior portion of each body; therefore, the effect of weight, after the compression of the soft tissues, the intervertebral discs in particular, would be a rotation of the bones in the path of least resistance, or, away from the line of stress, toward the convexity of the curve.

In functional curvature the bodies of the vertebræ have rotated to the concavity of the curve; in structural curvature, they have rotated to the convexity of the curve. The transverse processes have taken part in the revolution of the vertebra until in scoliosis upon the side of the convexity may be found the high side, upon the concavity the low side. As the transition from functional to structural takes place, as the bodies are turning, there comes a time when the body of any particular vertebra is directly in front, antero-posteriorly, of the spinous process. The vertebra itself shows a sidetilting to the right when the concavity is on the right, or expressed more exactly, a line erected perpendicularly to the upper surface of the body of the vertebra would

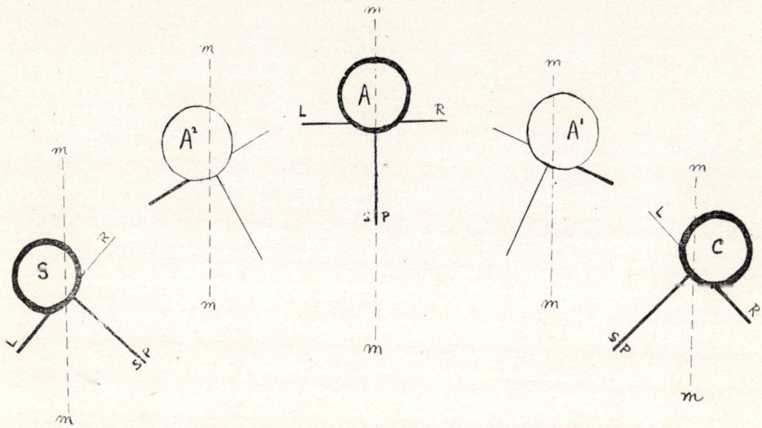

FIG. 11.—The rotation of the vertebræ from the functional stage F to the structural stage S, passes through the intermediary stages A1, A, A2. S. P. spinous process; L, left transverse process; R, right transverse process; M-M, antero-posterior line projected from the axis of rotation of each vertebra when in its normal position.

project upward and to the right. At this place in the rotation of the vertebra, there is no undue prominence of either transverse process, so that it is impossible to distinguish a high side and a low side. This stage of curvature may be named the transitional, a stage midway between functional and structural wherein there is yet no change in the shape of the bones. A curvature, as indicated by the line of spinous processes exists but without the other differentiating signs. In examining a patient with curvature, of which the high side is difficult to determine, it is safe to suspect that the curvature is in the transitional stage and that the bodies are in the process of turning toward the convexity. The prognosis

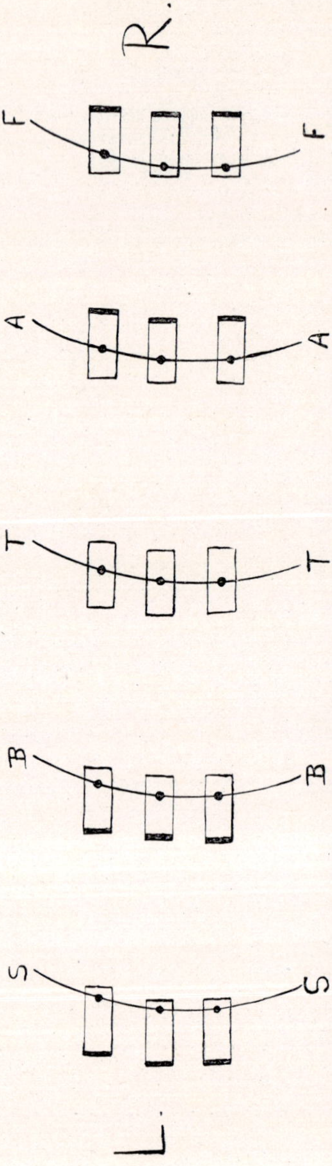

FIG. 12.—The lines from F-F to S-S represent the line of spinous processes in a curvature progressing from the functional stage to scoliosis. The rectangles represent the vertebral bodies, the round dots the spinous processes. The line T-T represents bodies and spinous processes in the transitional stage.

in such a case would be the same as for a case with moderate scoliosis except in one class of cases, those with flexible spines at a time when the vertebral bodies have not rotated beyond a plane parallel with the sagital plane of the body. The mechanical principle in the treatment of such a case would be to turn the curvature back to the functional stage while building up the general vitality and removing the cause, and then correct the functional curve by the usual process.

That few cases are found in the transitional stage is due to the fact that little attention is paid to a lack of symmetry appearing in the growing child or adolescent. Much is left to chance by parents and guardians. It has been the popular idea that children will outgrow defects for nature will overcome every ill, overlooking the fact that habit is ten times stronger than nature. School boards insist upon examining a child's eyes, ears, nose, and throat, but ask no privilege in regard to his spine, nor even suggest to parents the advisability of consulting a physician until the case with an easily rectified functional curvature has progressed into the almost incurable stage of scoliosis.

Total functional curves most frequently change to total scolioses, but it is common for a double curve to be formed in this change, with a small percentage of cases changing to scolioses of limited extent, oftenest with the resulting curve in the dorsal area.

Following the transitional stage begins true scoliosis, with a change in the shape of the vertebræ, due to the fact that bone under pressure is not markedly resistant.[1] Bone is plastic, a quality which as Wolff of Berlin has shown, causes it to change in response to functional demands. Wolff's law is as follows: "Every change in the formation and function of bones, or of their function alone, is followed by certain definite changes in their internal structure and equally definite secondary alterations of their external conformation in accordance with mathematical laws."

1. A study of the resistance of bone and of the soft tissues offers some strange deductions, namely, that bone is less resistant than is generally supposed and soft tissues more resistant. There seems no limit to the amount of deformity possible in any particular bone while on the other hand the resistance of soft tissues may set a limit to the extent of the osseous deformity and contrariwise often is the means by which it is perpetuated as for example adaptive shortening or contracture of muscles on the concavity of a lateral spinal curvature.

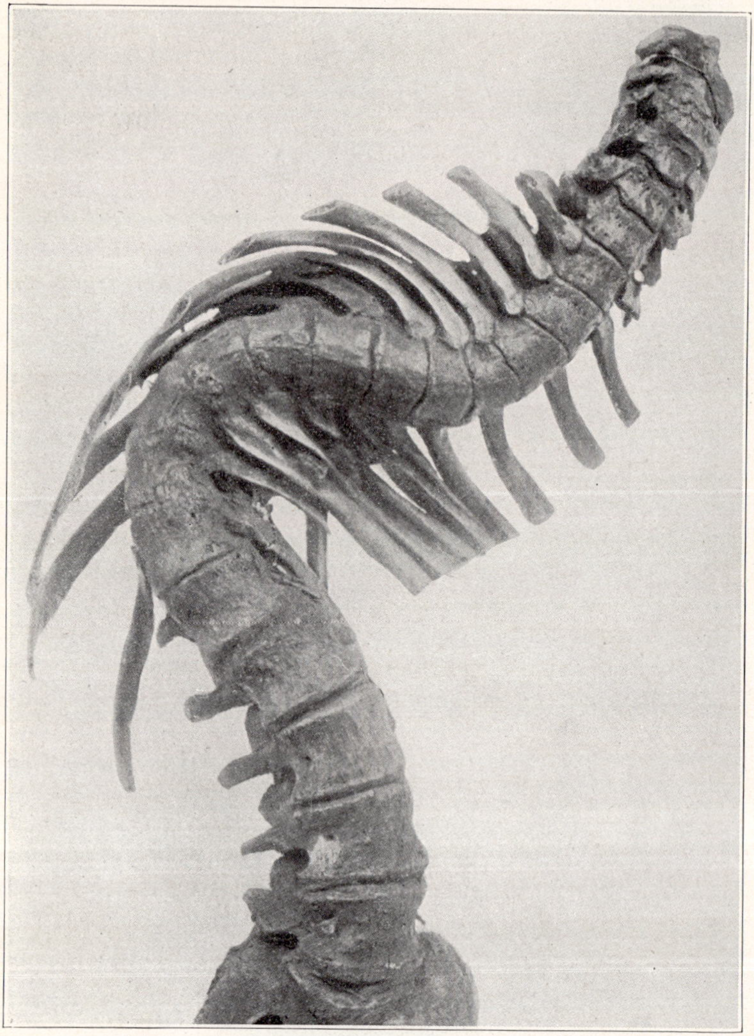

FIG. 13.—Scoliotic spine. (J. S. K. Smith).

Following this rule of plasticity Wolff[1] further explains: "According to this reasoning, deformities are nothing less than the result of the transformations which the external form of bones or joints undergoes in accommodating itself to faulty demands. It must be self-evident that that which is pathological is only the altered static requirement, the abnormal mechanical function. Far from being really pathological the deformity is the only suitable or even possible form by means of which bone or joint can withstand the altered forces bearing upon it; it is nature's way of securing the greatest possible service and strength under new conditions with the use of the least possible amount of material.

"In the absence of an abnormal softness of bone, the body of a vertebra may lose height on the concave side and gain the same on the convex side through the 'tropic stimulus of function' purely; being simply an accommodation to the diminished space on the concave side and increased room at the convexity and the change of mechanical conditions consequent thereupon."[2]

The pathological effects occuring in scoliosis vary in degree from mere asymmetry to marked distortion. The first effect comes in the vertebræ themselves. At the apex of the curve the bodies of the vertebræ become wedge-shaped, with the base of the wedge between the lateral and ventral surfaces of the body on the concavity of the curve; with the apex of the wedge between the posterior and lateral surfaces of the body on the convexity of the curve. The spinous processes in the lumbar region are deflected toward the concavity; in the dorsal area while turned toward the concavity, they tend to be deflected at the tip downward and toward the convexity. The vertebræ between the apices of the curves and the normal part are oblique in character, the upper and lower surfaces sliding upon each other. Due to the crowding together of the articular processes on the side of the concavity, there is an increase in their size, while on the convexity from the separation of the pedicles, they are smaller and higher. In many specimens, synostoses are found between the joints on the concavity with some ossification of their ligaments.

---

1. Die Lehre von der functionellen Pathogenese der Deformitæten, Archiv. fur klinische Chirurgie, Bd. liii., H. 4.

2. Translation more complete in Whitman's "Orthopedic Surgery," 4th Edit., page 242.

The ligamentous changes correspond to the osseous changes. On the side of the concavity the anterior longitudinal and lateral spinal ligaments are thicker and shorter than in the normal flexible spine. On the convexity they are thinned, longer, and somewhat atrophied.

Muscular changes are easily palpated. Because of the rigidity which comes early in cases of scoliosis, there is a general atrophy

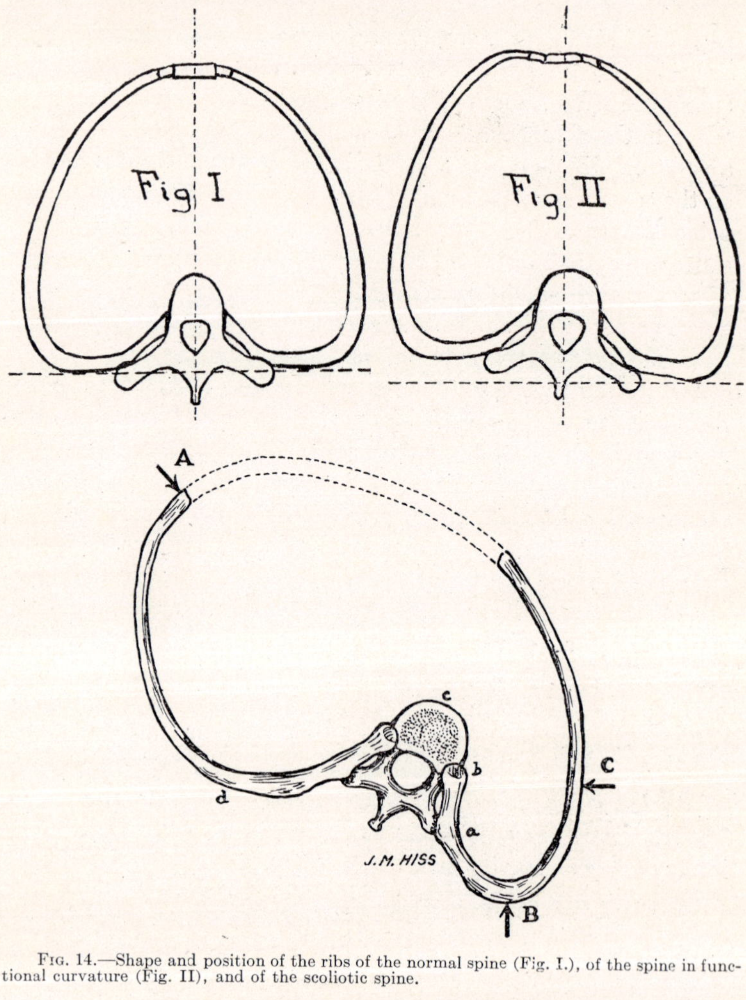

FIG. 14.—Shape and position of the ribs of the normal spine (Fig. I.), of the spine in functional curvature (Fig. II), and of the scoliotic spine.

of the muscles of the back from lack of use. On the concave side a fibrous degeneration is a frequent condition; on the convex side there is a thinning and wasting of muscle tissue.

Severe cases are characterized by great deformities in other osseous structures beside the spine. Some of these changes are marked, especially in the ribs, which by the influence of the rotation of the vertebral bodies and the longitudinal tension of the spinal muscles, are not only changed in their relation to other bones, but show structural changes in angularity, which on the side of the convexity shows a marked increase, throwing the scapula backward so that it often appears to be larger than its fellow; from the angle forward to their costal extremities these ribs have less than the normal curve, are much more oblique, and are spread farther apart. On the concavity the angles are straightened, the shafts present an increased curve, are more horizontal, and closer together. The scapula on the concavity lies close to the thorax.

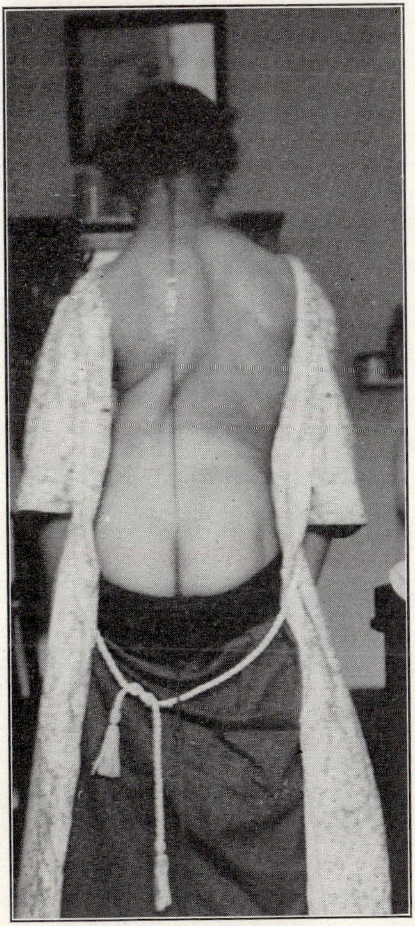

FIG. 15.—Scoliosis. (Laughlin).

The sternum and clavicle show slight changes in conformation. The pelvis in its deformities is like the thorax but much less in degree.

The appearance of the patient with a structural curvature varies with the intensity of the curve, and with the area involved. Lumbar scolioses are characterized by less deformity than presented by other areas. The apparently larger hip and the depth of waist-line on the concave side and the displacement of the trunk to the convexity are the principle signs of the lumbar curvature. Diagnosis rests upon the presence of the high side upon the convexity. The patient in bending over loses none of the appearance of curvature, and the high side persists upon the convexity.

It must not be forgotten that lumbar rotation is less than dorsal rotation, being always secondary to side-bending, therefore curvatures which might appear to be slight in that region may in reality be severe.

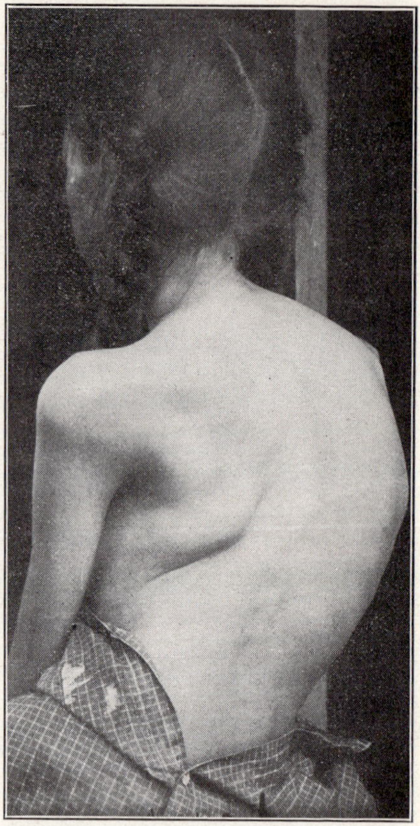

FIG. 16.—Incurable Scoliosis. (Laughlin).

A case of total scoliosis has the same signs as a lumbar curve, with the additional sign of the high shoulder on the convexity and changes in the lower ribs. Dorsal scoliosis presents the most marked deformities. A patient with a dorsal scoliosis convex to the left presents this picture: the thorax as a whole is displaced to the left; the left arm hangs farther from the side than the right arm; the waist-line on the left is flattened, on the right deeper; the contour of the chest is changed anteriorly and the longest diameter is an oblique antero-posterior line from the left scapula to the right nipple. The line of spinous processes is no guide to

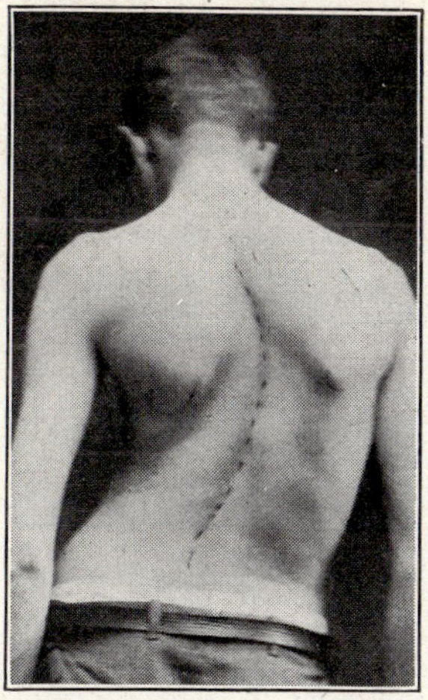

FIG. 17.—Scoliosis, right dorsal primary, left lumbar secondary. (Laughlin).

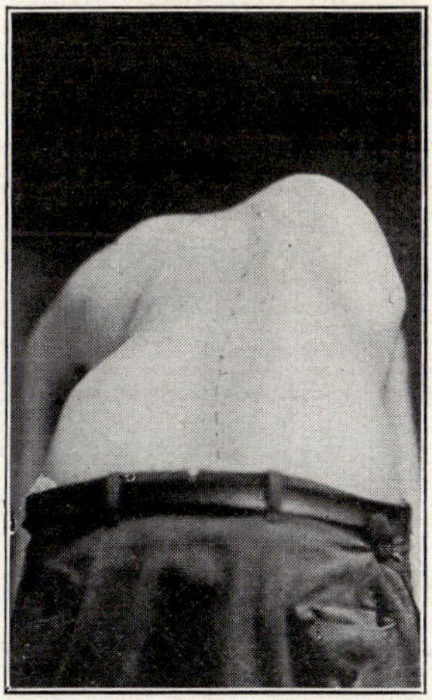

FIG. 18.—Same patient in flexion, showing high side on the convexity. (Laughlin).

the amount of rotation present in the vertebral bodies for the bodies in structural curvature move farther from the sagital plane than the spines.

Compound structural curvatures combine the features of the simple scolioses. They are more frequent than any other class, occurring in thirty percent of all cases. Scolioses may change

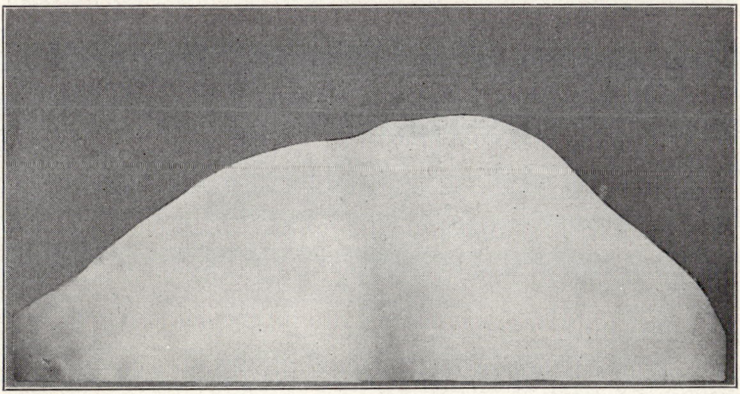

FIG. 19.—Lumbar scoliosis, showing high side on the convexity.

from one clinical type to another in the course of years. Total curves change to compound curves oftenest, and compensatory curves follow all types. Schulthess tabulated over one thousand cases in the order of their coming for treatment and found the relative frequency of certain types as follows:

Compound scoliosis	30 percent
Dorsolumbar . .	20 "
Dorsal	19 "
Total	15 "
Lumbar	11 "
Cervicodorsal .	3 "

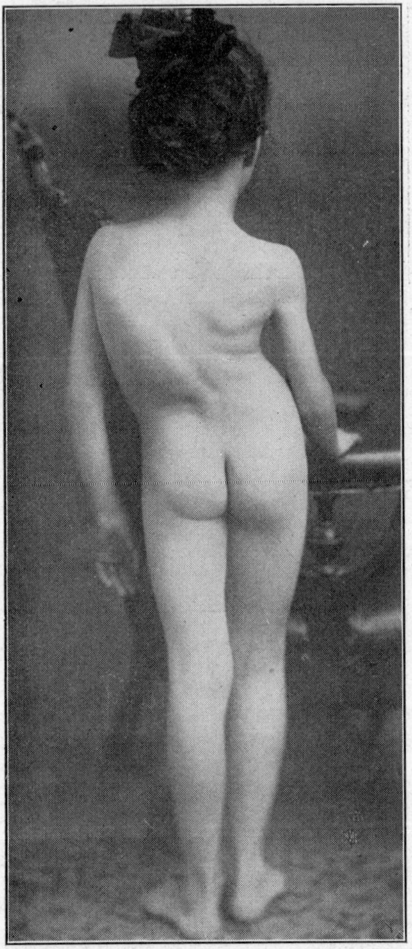

FIG. 20.—Left dorsal scoliosis from anterior poliomyelitis. (Laughlin.)

The patients who have scoliosis do not manifest any symptoms directly resulting from the condition unless the case belongs to the severe type when pain is often complained of and is probably due to strain from altered muscular or ligamentous tension, pressure from distorted ribs upon nerve fibres, or as a neurasthenic symptom of lowered vitality and decreased resistance to ordinary irritations.

In consequence of the alteration in the shape of the thorax there are noticeable pressure effects upon the viscera with pathological conditions following. The chest diameter on the convex

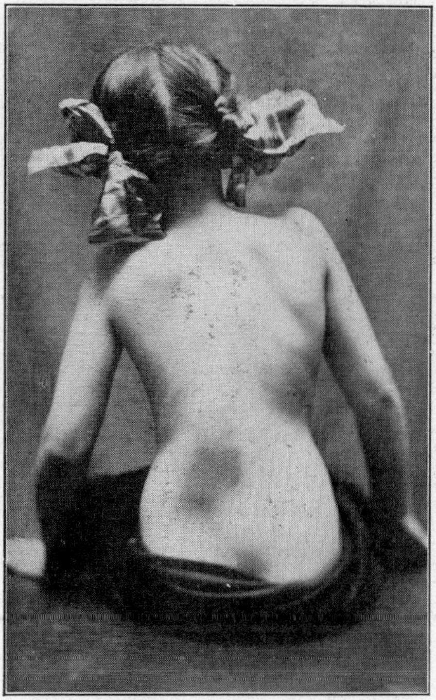

FIG. 21.—Same patient as Fig. 20. Scoliosis corrected with two casts, during six months of treatment. (Laughlin).

side is much reduced and in consequence there is less lung capacity. Anemia may be a secondary effect. The heart may suffer displacement. Venous dilatation and cardiac hypertrophy may be found due to the difficulty with which the heart pumps the blood through the lungs in the effort to ærate it.

The abdominal contents on account of the restriction of space suffer from the crowding and displacement. Diseases in the liver, kidneys, spleen, intestines, and stomach, in patients of the scoliotic type, are undoubtedly due to spinal conditions and thoracic deformities.

TREATMENT

The problem presented by any case of structural curvature is the overcoming of bone deformity and as such belongs properly

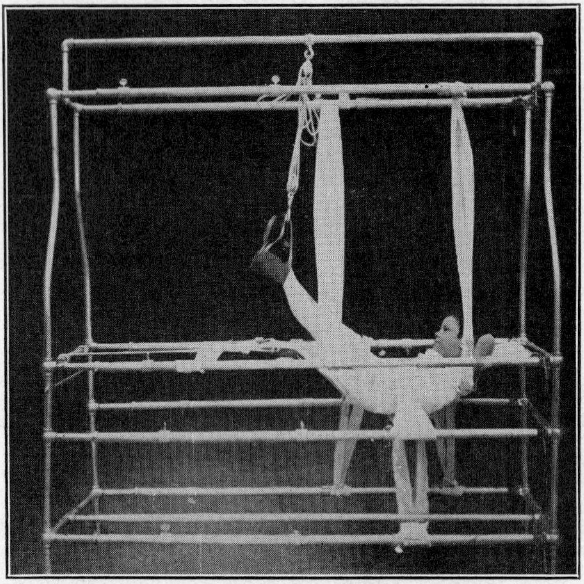

FIG. 22.—The Abbott frame in position for application of a cast in a case of right thoracic scoliosis. (Laughlin.)

to orthopedic surgery. For four thousand years scoliosis has been regarded as a muscle problem and in consequence the history of its treatment is largely one of failure.

The first logically sound solution of the problem was offered by the recent studies of Lovett and others into the mechanics of the spine. Sidebending and rotation had not been understood and until the principle of these movements was discovered and applied to the treatment of curvature, advance was impossible.

Less than a decade ago a Portland orthopedist, E. C. Abbott, offered the first truly mechanical foundation for correction of the deviation. Its principle is physiological production of sidebending-rotation in a position which shall carry the bodies of the vertebræ to the convexity and to maintain them in this position until the bones shall have changed their shape back toward the normal.

The process of application is as follows:

I. The position of flexion.—The patient lies in a hammock or canvas sling which hangs in a gas-pipe frame. (Fig. 22.) The hammock is cut on the bias so that beneath the shoulder on the concavity there shall be more room.

II. The pelvis is fixed by straps fastened to a lateral arm of the frame, on the side of the convexity. A similar strap pulls up the low shoulder, to stretch the concavity and raise the shoulder. A strap is put around the thorax at the convexity of the curvature and fastened to a lateral arm of the frame on the side of the concavity so that it can be pulled laterally until sidebending has been given the convexity.

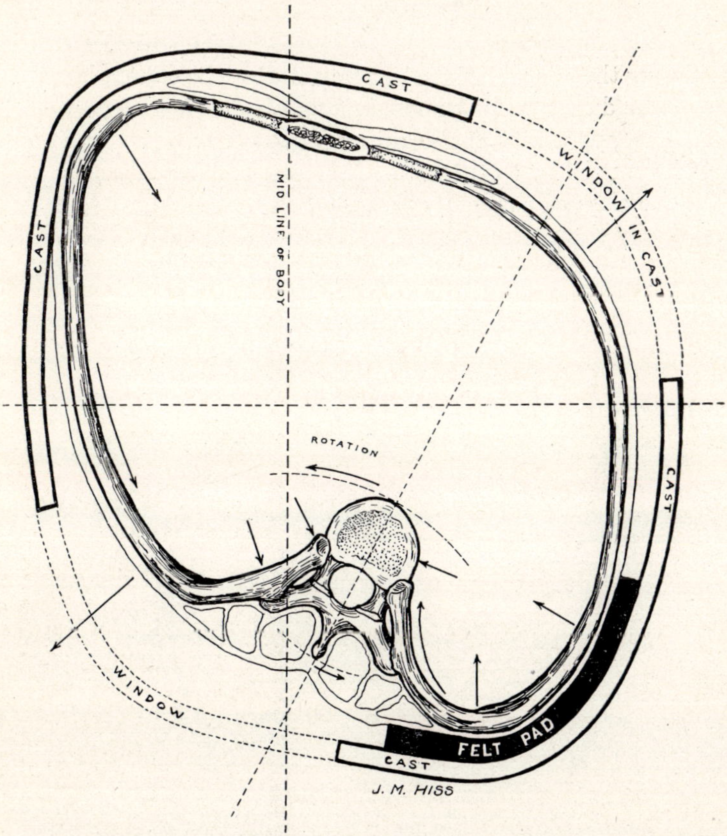

Fig. 23.—The deformity of the thorax in scoliosis. The holes which should be cut in the cast and the location for extra pressure by felt pads are indicated. The arrows show the directions of the various forces. (Laughlin.)

III. Immobilization is now made by the application of a plaster of Paris cast.

IV. To assist in the rotation of the vertebræ, pressure is applied over the angles of the ribs on the convexity with reinforcement diagonally across on the ventral surface by the insertion of pads from time to time. Over the angles of the ribs on the concavity and diagonally across in front openings are made in the cast so that respiration may cause the ribs to bulge and regain their normal shape.

V. Over-correction is the last step for it is necessary to make permanent the changes wrought by the application of the casts. It is maintained until the thorax returns to its normal contour. Following the removal of the last plaster cast, the patient is placed for a time during waking hours in a celluloid or leather jacket, so that an opportunity for acquiring strength may be given the muscles wasted by the pressure of the cast and from disuse.

The class of patients who are cured by the Abbott cast are principally those with the simple forms of scoliosis or, better, the long total or dorsal types. Very few double scolioses are bene-

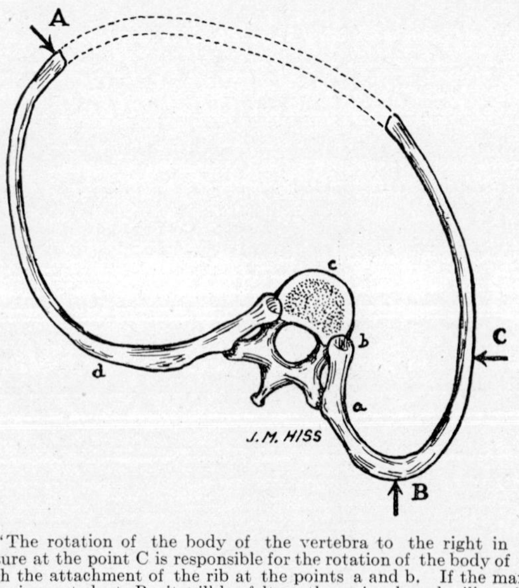

FIG. 24.—"The rotation of the body of the vertebra to the right in a right dorsal scoliosis. Pressure at the point C is responsible for the rotation of the body of the vertebra to the right through the attachment of the rib at the points a and b. If the maximum of pressure in correction is exerted at B, it will be felt at the point b and will tend to reduce the rotation." (Laughlin.)

fitted. Casts in these cases are applied for what seems to have been the primary curve; after its correction the compensatory or secondary curve would naturally disappear; if it did not, after time had been given for the secondary curve to be determined as to its permanent character, it should receive appropriate treatment.

The patients must be well-nourished children or young adults. Frail children or very young children are not suitable patients for confinement in plaster casts. In the very young, it is sometimes possible with the changes incident to growing bone to accomplish correction by leather jackets or other appliances.

Those patients who have marked dorsal kyphoses with lateral deformitiy are not much helped for the reason that when the vertebræ are immobilized in flexion, there is already all the forward bending the vertebræ will stand, and without flexion beyond that held in the curvature, the articular processes could not be "unlocked," nor the tension of the intervertebral discs changed, both of which are essential to correction of vertebral lesions singly or in groups.

Osteopathic treatment, aside from that outlined above, given by the orthopedic specialists of our school of practice, should be given before the cast operation and after it. It should be in the nature of a general treatment, which the author holds is putting the spinal joints through their normal movements as far as possible. Flexibility is indispensable to the early correction of scoliosis by cast. Movements of flexion and extension and torsion away from the convexity, are indicated.

Following the removal of the plaster cast, and while the patient is wearing the celluloid one, treatment should be given for the upbuilding of muscle strength and increased vitality of the patient. As soon as the jackets are left off, the patient should be given exercises strictly under the direction of the physician for the development of muscular strength throughout the body. The same movements that have been before recommended in the after-treatment of functional curvature may be given. In addition special attention should be given to the leg and thigh muscles so that the patient may be able to stand and walk without fatigue; to the chest-expanding muscles to increase respiratory capacity;

to the muscles of vertebroscapular attachment so that the shoulder girdles may be supported with comfort; to the abdominal and spinal muscles to strengthen the spine, and to the cervical area for the easy carriage of the head. The field is a large one for the osteopathist. He best of all classes of physicians is fitted for this work.

The detail of the Abbott method has not been given. The reader is referred to the excellent monograph of Dr. George M. Laughlin, reprinted from the "Journal of Osteopathy," for March, 1914, for the technique of this method and the results obtained.

In regard to the treatment that has been accorded these cases by the gymnastic method, it seems advisable to state that the dangers are greater than any possible good that could be derived therefrom. Robert W. Lovett[1] has covered this point well, as follows:

"Not only may gymnastics in moderate and severe structural scoliosis fail to do good, but they frequently do serious harm for the following reason: scoliosis of this grade soon results in a stiffening of the affected region of the spine. If efficient gymnastics are given, the spine is speedily rendered more flexible and if it is so rendered and not supported at once it will sink into a worse position than before and the curve will be increased."

1. Lovett, ibid, page 127, second paragraph.

CHAPTER IV.

FLEXION AND EXTENSION LESIONS

FLEXION LESIONS

A flexion lesion is a subluxation, or an immobilization, of a vertebral articulation in the position of flexion.

It is not abnormal for any spinal joint at some period in the life of the individual to assume the position characteristic of a flexion lesion, but it is abnormal at any time for that joint to become immobilized in flexion. Immobilization may be defined as fixation and differs from the static position of rest in the pathological changes that have taken place in the supporting and surrounding tissues and also in the fact that it is mechanically inert. Its restoration to function depends upon the overcoming of physiological reactions and pathological restrictions. Occasionally these readjustments are spontaneous.

From the study of the normal movement of flexion, the anatomical relations present in lesion may be deduced:

Spinous process.—Separated from the one below, approximated to the one above.

Facets.—Parts of the articular surfaces in apposition.

Body.—Slightly anterior at the anterior inferior margin.

Disc.—Compresssed anteriorly and stretched somewhat posteriorly.

Ligaments.

I. Stretched, thinned, and atrophied
  - a. Posterior longitudinal.
  - b. Flava.
  - c. Supraspinous.
  - d. Interspionous.
  - e. Intertransverse.

II. Relaxed and thickened
  - a. Anterior longitudinal.

Intervertebral foramina.—Increased in size above, decreased below.[1]

1. The separation of the pedicles of the vertebra in lesion and of the one below is meant. In fact, the foramina are ultimately decreased in size by the deposition of connective tissue, the result of the inflammatory changes that take place while the lesion is in the acute stage.

Muscles.—Fasciculi of the extensor muscules of that area stretched and atrophied; corresponding muscles of flexion contracted.

The determination of a flexion lesion is made by palpation.[1] In the early literature of osteopathy the flexion lesion was called posterior, for the reason that the spinous process of the vertebra in lesion appears more prominent than adjacent ones. The reason for this prominence is due to the separation of its tip from

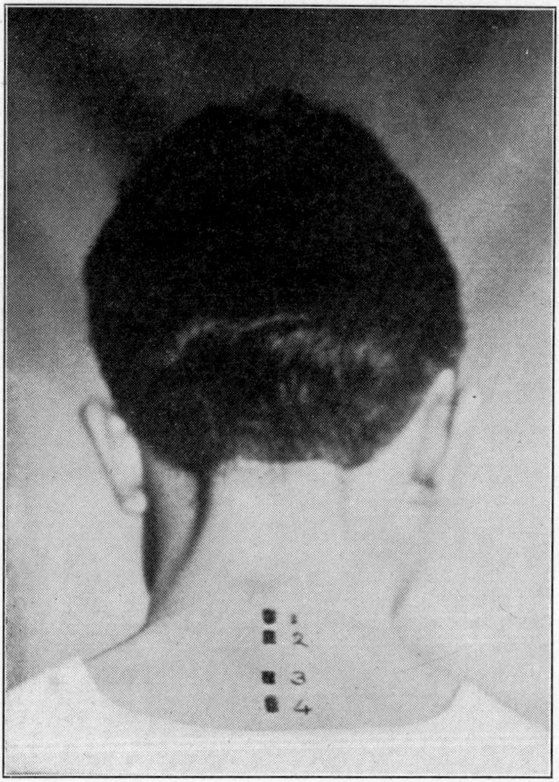

FIG. 25.—The appearance of the spinous processes when a flexion lesion is present in the second-third thoracic articulation.

1. It should be required of every patient coming for examination that he bare his spine for inspection and palpation. In no other way can an accurate diagnosis be made.

that of the spinous process below, throwing the upper of the two into relief in the plane of the back. In the examination of a patient prominences should be noted and careful palpation made to determine whether or not they are indicative of flexion lesions. A spinous process may be posterior in relation to the general line of spinous processes and yet not be the sign of a flexion lesion. Such processes are usually anomalous conditions, the spinous process being longer than its fellows and longer than that of the normal vertebra. THE PROOF OF LESION IS LOSS OF FUNCTION, RESTRICTED MOTION.

EXPERIMENTAL PALPATION, A.—Ask the patient, B, to sit upon a stool, while O stands beside him. B's spine should be bare.[1] Let O pass his fingers down the row of upper thoracic spinous processes until he finds the one which seems more prominent than the others. Let us assume that it is the sixth thoracic. Let O place the ball of his forefinger between the fifth and sixth spinous processes and the ball of the second finger between the sixth and seventh. O should compare the distance between these spinous processes. If the sixth is in flexion lesion, its spine will be farther from the seventh than from the fifth. Let O compare also the distance between adjacent spinous processes above and below.

Let O place his other hand upon B's head and move it forward strongly. In the normal spine, or the spine having a sixth thoracic vertebra with a long process, there will be increased separation between the spinous processes, and the movement in separation

---

1. Osteopathic diagnosis rests largely upon the difficult art of palpation. It is that part of the student's preparation which should be emphasized from the outset. Since people vary physically to the degree that one may say when the problem under consideration is technique, that every human being is a law unto himself, it may be best to outline what I think should be the course of private study for each student who is beginning this work.

The spine of the living model is indispensable to the student. He should select at first a model who is about twenty years of age, in good health, and as far as possible one who has no lesions. By placing the balls of his fingers between every two spinous processes, he may palpate the change in their relations while the subject makes the normal movements of the spine. As soon as the student feels that he has acquired the ability to detect movement in the spinal articulations of the various areas in this subject, he should select models who have spines less easily palpated, as those who are old, prematurely rigid, obese, over-muscular, and hypermobile. With the advance in the work, while he is studying lesions, he should ask the privilege of examining the spines of as many people as would be interested in assisting him to cultivate his sense of touch. C. P. McConnell says "Educated fingers do not come by chance but only by the hardest kind of labor and effort." He thinks also that six to nine months are necessary for this foundation. See "The Journal of the A. O. A." for March, 1913, page 417.

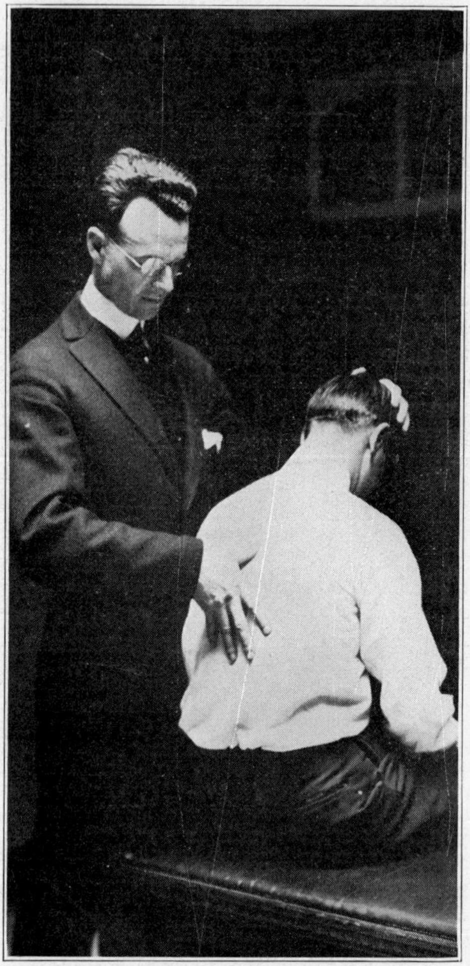

FIG. 26.—Manner of palpating for flexion and extension lesions of the thoracic area. The hand upon the head uses it as a lever to produce movement in the thoracic region. The thumb between the spinous processes determines the presence or absence of motion.

will be easily detected. If a flexion lesion is present, there will be no change in the separation of the sixth and seventh. Let O then carry B's head backward strongly in extension, whereupon if lesion is not present, the spinous process of the sixth will approximate that of the seventh. If the sixth is in flexion lesion, there will be no change in the relative distance between the spinous processes.

From the above experimental palpation, the terms of the diagnosis of a flexion lesion may be stated:

THE SPINOUS PROCESS OF A VERTEBRA IN FLEXION LESION IS SEPARATED FROM THE SPINOUS PROCESS OF THE VERTEBRA BELOW AND ANY MOVEMENT OF THAT AREA OF THE SPINE DOES NOT CHANGE THE AMOUNT OF SEPARATION BETWEEN THE TWO PROCESSES.

EXPERIMENTAL PALPATION, B.—Since flexion lesions of the lumbar area are sometimes difficult to diagnose with the patient seated upon a stool, let the patient, B, who is supposed to have a flexion lesion of the fourth lumbar vertebra, lie upon his left side upon the operating table, facing O who stands beside the table. O flexes B's knees and places them against O's abdomen, while he holds B firmly upon the table by placing his right hand over the dorsolumbar area of his back. O places the finger tips of his left hand along the spinous processes of B's lumbar area with the purpose of finding the prominent fourth lumbar spinous process and of comparing the distance between it and the adjacent spinous processes. If the fourth is in flexion lesion, its spinous

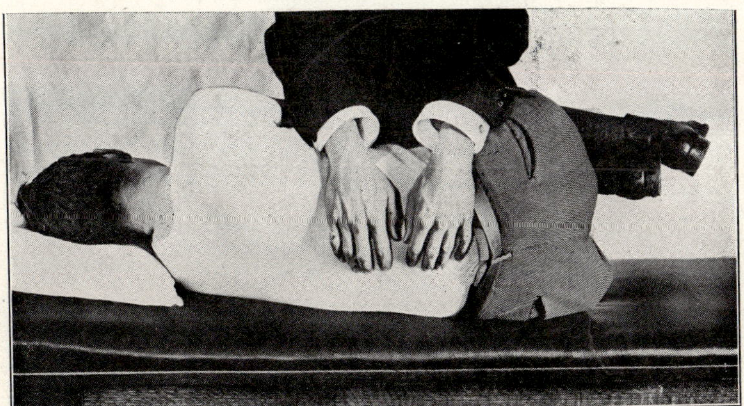

FIG. 27.—Manner of palpating for the detection of flexion and extension lesions of the lumbar area.

process would be farther from the fifth than from the third. By shifting his weight from one foot to the other, at the same time maintaining firm pressure with his right hand upon B's spine, O may produce flexion and extension in B's lumbar area and detect the presence or absence of motion in those joints. If the palpating finger finds separation and restricted motion in the fourth-fifth interspace, then the diagnosis of flexion lesion is confirmed.

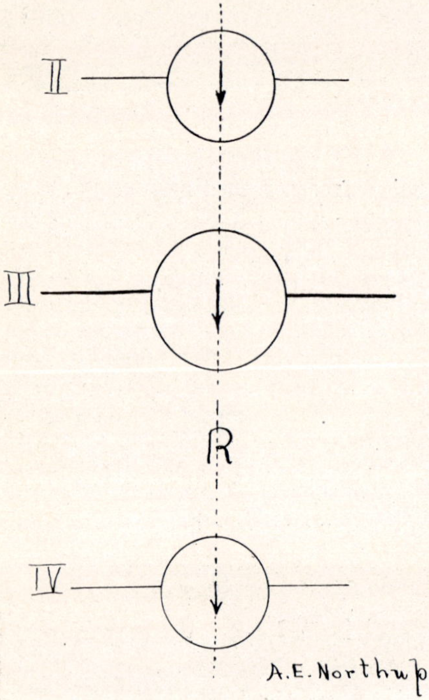

FIG. 28.—Schematic drawing to illustrate the separation of spinous processes in the case of a flexion lesion of the third-fourth lumbar articulation. The larger size of the circle, indicating the spinous process of the third, represents its prominence as seen when looking at the back. In the interspace R, motion is found restricted.

Differential diagnosis will substantiate preliminary diagnosis and should be a part of every routine examination. Flexion lesions are to be differentiated from

1. Extension lesion of the vertebra below by restricted motion in the interspace where there is separation of spinous processes and free motion in the interspace where there is an approximation of spinous processes.

2. The anomalous condition of a fourth lumbar vertebra[1] with a long spinous process which would be determined by the presence of movement in the third-fourth and fourth-fifth joints.

3. The anomalous condition of a short spinous process of an adjacent vertebra determined by the presence of motion in the joints above and below.

Flexion lesions are most commonly the result of strain. An individual bending forward in as much flexion as his spine will permit, is acted upon by a superior force with the result that one

1. The spinous process of the fourth lumbar vertebra is frequently longer than normal, while the fifth lumbar has normally the shortest spinous process among the lumbars. The third is mentioned by some writers as the one having the thickest spinous process.

or more of the spinal articulations are forced into greater flexion, in reality into subluxation, wherein the articulating surfaces remain but slightly apposed. Upon resuming the upright position, all of the spinal joints, save those injured, return to the normal. Examination of the lesioned articulations would reveal the fact that ligaments, whose purpose has been not only to connect bones but to limit motion in the joint, have been unduly stretched and will quickly show the effects of injury, congestion and subsequently atrophy, thinning, and sometimes calcareous deposit.

Strain usually occurs suddenly and unexpectedly, by accident, blows, falls, or the lifting of heavy weights. Certain areas are prone to these lesions, especially the cervicodorsal and dorsolumbar junctions due to the restricted mobility of the thoracic region, and the greater freedom of motion in the cervical and lumbar areas. The lumbar region[1] is also liable to these lesions because upon that area of the spine rests the greatest amount of superincumbent weight.

Sometimes by gradual production are flexion lesions formed. Muscular insufficiency is the source of the final result. The first cause may be infection, toxin, or any one of many agencies setting up an irritation in or about the joint, from which the individual seeks relief by carrying the spine uneasily in flexion. The fasciculi of the extensor muscles are stretched and unbalance is present. The flexors hold what they have gained and in time the same amount of change has taken place in the spinal joint that might have been occasioned by a sudden expenditure of force. Injuries to the muscle mass of any of the extensors or weakness from other cause, or irritations causing contractions of flexors, would act in the same manner to assist in the production of a flexion lesion. Group lesions are always of gradual production.

CORRECTIVE MOVEMENTS

The Principle of Correction for flexion lesions is extension.

1. Flexion lumbar lesions are etiologic in causing pelvic, bladder, and rectal disorders. Constipation of the large intestine may often be traced directly to such a lesion and leucorrhea is a common symptom of a fifth lumbar flexion lesion.

GENERAL RULES.—THE ARTICULATING SURFACES MUST RETRACE THE PATH THEY TOOK IN THEIR DISPLACEMENT. It has been well said that it requires but a little force at exactly the right angle to produce a lesion and conversely that a little force applied in exactly the right direction will reduce a subluxation.[1]

There are two methods commonly employed by osteopathists in the correction of lesions the older of which is the traction method, the later the direct method or thrust.[2] Those who employ the traction method secure the relaxation of the tissues about the articulation by what has been termed exaggeration of the lesion, a motion in the direction of the forcible movement which produced the lesion, as if its purpose were to increase the deformity. C. P. McConnell states that this disengages the tissues that are holding the parts in the abnormal position. It is more than probable that the effectiveness of this procedure is due to the physiological reaction that is set up in those tissues which have the power of contractility, the flava ligaments and the extensor muscle fasciculi in the case of the lesions under discussion. The exaggeration is held, traction made upon the joint, replacement initiated and then completed by reversal of the forces.[3]

The direct method consists in the application of a precisely directed force toward a bony prominence during the process of putting the articulation in lesion through the spinal movement which is the reversal of that which produced the lesion. Relaxation of restraining tissues is secured by the corrective movements preliminary to adjustment. It avoids the expenditure of force often essential to the successful use of traction.

1. CHIN-RAISING MOVEMENT.—A patient, B, is assumed to have a flexion lesion of the second thoracic. Let the patient sit upon a stool while O stands at his left side. O places B's chin in the bend of his elbow, passing the forearm up beside B's cheek and resting the hand lightly on his head. O places the hypothenar eminence of his right hand against the spinous process of the second thoracic vertebra, the palm of the hand resting against the back of B's

1. Statement of Dr. Ethel Louise Burner, Bloomington, Ill.

2. The term "direct" is preferred for the reason that the imitators of osteopathy have given to the word "thrust" an objectionable meaning of harshness.

3. This method is the more difficult of the two and for the instruction of students does not find favor with the author.

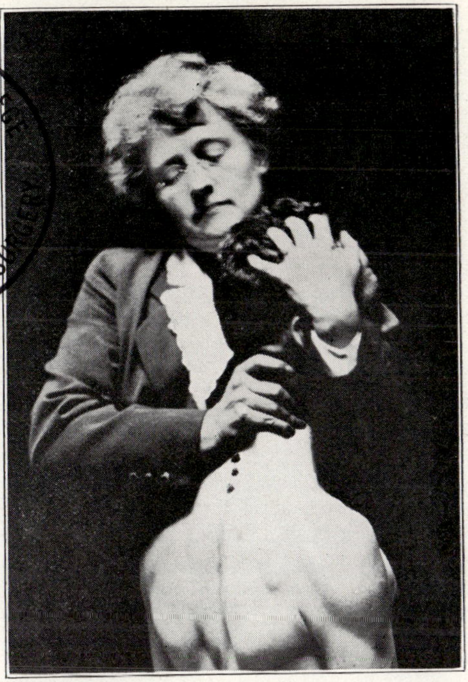

Fig. 29.—Illustrating the chin-raising movement.

neck, the thumb and forefinger spread below B's occiput. O puts firm pressure against the point of attack, the spinous process, maintains the palm of his hand flat to prevent extension in the cervical region, holds the outspread thumb and finger as a fulcrum against which by raising the left elbow the head may be carried backward in extension. The movement is repeated until relaxation is secured, when with a little additional force at the limit of extension adjustment is made.

This movement is corrective for flexion lesions from the seventh cervical to the fourth thoracic usually.

II. Supine Movement—The patient, B, is assumed to be acutely ill and suffering from conditions that are aggravated by a flexion lesion of the fifth thoracic. B lies supine with his arms over his head. O bends over him and places his hands under B's back crossing the forefingers upon the spinous process of the fifth thoracic. B is asked to inhale slowly and then exhale in the same manner, the purpose of this being to distract his attention and to secure relaxation. During his expiration O lifts up against the spinous process of the vertebra in lesion and holds the pressure until B inhales again. After several repetitions, at the conclusion of expiration, with a sudden slight increase of force directed against the spinous process anteriorly and downward towards B's feet, the lesion is adjusted.

This movement is corrective for flexion lesions from the second to seventh dorsal inclusive.

III. ROCKING MOVEMENT.—B is assumed to have a flexion lesion of the seventh thoracic. He sits upon a stool or the table, depending upon the height of himself and his physician. He clasps his arms across his shoulders and leans them against O's chest. O passes his arms under B's axillæ and around his back until he can place one or more fingers strongly over the spinous process of the vertebra in lesion. O rocks B forward and backward in flexion and extension until relaxation is secured and then with a slight additional force directed against the spinous process anteriorly and downward, the lesion is adjusted. If the patient is of light weight, traction may be very easily used with this movement at the moment just before adjustment.

This movement is effective for the correction of lesions from the third to the ninth thoracic inclusive and may be used in the treatment of patients who are convalescent after acute illness.

IV. STOOL-AND-ELBOW MOVEMENT.—Let B sit upon a stool and clasp his arms across his shoulders. O stands to B's left and passes his left forearm under B's arms to support him and also to lift the upper part of his body as a lever. O places his right elbow against the spinous process of the dorsal vertebra in flexion lesion, and carries his forearm up against B's back and rests the palm of the hand upon his head to assist in producing extension at the required time. B rests much of his weight upon O's left arm and O carries B forward in greater flexion and then raises B's arms and gradually carries his thoracic area back in extension until the movement reaches the joint in lesion. At the same time he is placing pressure against the spinous process of the lesioned vertebra through his elbow. The movement is repeated until relaxation is complete, and then with slightly increased force adjustment is secured.

This movement may be used to correct flexion lesions from the fifth to the tenth thoracic vertebræ inclusive. In place of the elbow, pressure may be made against the point of attack with the thumb, a finger, or the hypothenar eminence.

V. CHEST FORWARD MOVEMENT.—The patient is supposed to have a flexion lesion of the eighth thoracic. Let him lie upon his face on the table and place his hands, palm downward, on the table beside his head. He is asked to raise his torso backward in extension and then is directed to carry the front of the thorax down toward the surface of the table for the purpose of localizing the extension. O may place his arm under B's chest to assist B

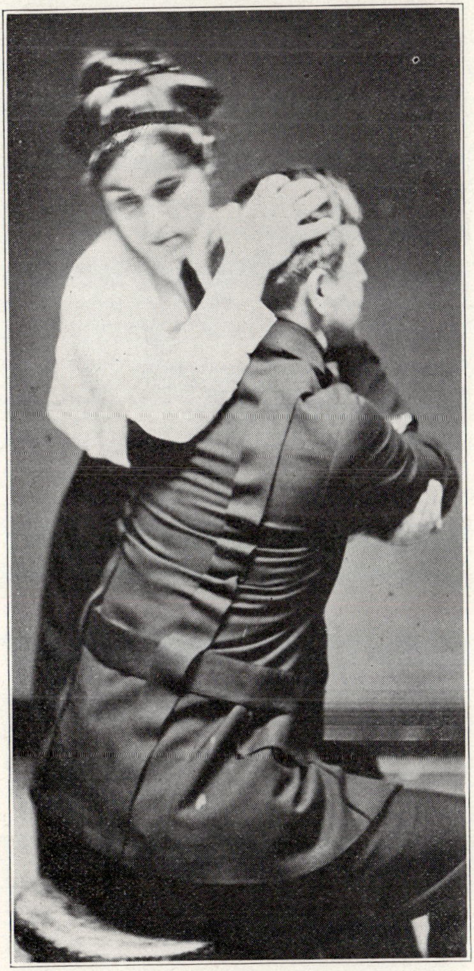

FIG. 30.—Illustrating the stool-and-elbow movement.

in raising himself from the table and to hold him firmly at the moment of adjustment. O places his other hand or thumb against the spinous process of the eighth dorsal and presses downward toward B's feet and anteriorly. After several repetitions[1] when relaxation has been secured, slight additional force at the point of lesion at the moment of greatest extension will adjust the subluxation.

This movement is corrective for flexion lesions from the fifth to the ninth thoracic inclusive.

VI. EXTENSION ASSISTING MOVEMENT.—The patient is assumed to have a flexion lesion of the third lumbar. He lies prone upon the table, places his hands as in the above movement and raises his torso backward in extension. O stands beside the table and assists B to raise his body by putting his arm across B's chest. O's other hand is placed against the spinous process of the third lumbar as a point of attack. When relaxation is complete, a well directed increase of force against the spinous process will adjust the lesion.

This movement may be used for the adjustment of flexion lesions from the eighth thoracic to the fifth lumbar inclusive.

VII. CIRCUMDUCTION EXTENSION MOVEMENT.[2]—B sits upon a stool facing O who stands in front of him, encircling him with his arms, and resting his fingers upon the spinous process of the first lumbar which is assumed to be in flexion lesion. B places his arms over O's shoulders, turns his face to one side and rests his head against O's shoulder. O carries B's body in circumduction backward, to the side, forward, to the other side, and repeats the movement. When he feels relaxation has been secured, he stops the movement in forward flexion and quickly carries B back in extension while he pulls anteriorly and downward upon the spinous process.

This movement is suitable for light-weight patients only and may be best given with traction just before the concluding direction of force against the spinous point of attack.

1. Patients respond differently to corrective movements. Some do not require a repetition of any movement. Others who do not voluntarily relax may need as many as five to eight repetitions of any given corrective movement before adjustment may be attempted.

2. A movement that has been used by many consists in lifting the thighs and pelvis of the patient, who lies prone upon the table, while pressure is made properly against the spinous process of the lesioned vertebra. The movement does not seem to me to be mechanically good for the reason that the superior articular facets of the vertebra below must be forced under the inferior facets of the vertebra above.

GROUP LESIONS

Group lesions may be corrected just as individual lesions by using less of final increase of force and more of extension for the purpose of stretching contractured flexor muscles. Rest in the prone position for frail patients is helpful when the patient's limbs are elevated by a roller of six inches' diameter placed beneath the knees or just above them. This brings extension upon the lumbar articulations and stretches the anterior longitudinal ligament and the discs anteriorly.

All patients should be advised to study their standing positions and sitting positions. The physician has not done his full duty to such a patient until he has explained the equilibrium of the erect body and advised them how they shall change faulty habits. It is as much a part of the routine examination as the finding of the lesion. Since group lesions are commonly the result of long continued faulty habit, it is not to be presumed that recovery may be made by the administration of a few corrective treatments. As a physician would give a sufferer from chronic nephritis a diet list, even so much it is necessary that a physician shall prescribe exercises when he finds the occasion. Nor should the physician fail to bring to the attention of the patient the part of the cure that devolves upon himself.[1] One is not justified in accepting a case when it is plain to be seen that the patient wilfully means not to concur in the plan proposed for overcoming the condition, which means that the cause must be removed before a cure can be made.[2]

AFTER-TREATMENT

Chronic flexion lesions may recur should the cause return. It is therefore best to institute a resistance form of treatment which

1. It has been my custom in examining patients for many years, especially since I have been examining for others to administer the treatment, to say to the patient having group lesions: "At least one-half of the cure of your condition depends upon the faithful performance on your part of the directions that shall be given you by your physician. You have no more right to expect the physician to cure you without your co-operation than the lazy poor man has to expect to be fed without toiling for the means wherewith to purchase food." The best results are obtainable after such plain statements as these.

2. It is axiomatic that the physician who inspires confidence in his patient is he who causes him to help himself. The most successful practices have been built by exactly such observances on the part of the physician.

shall be directed toward the strengthening of the extensor muscles whose tone has been lost. The patient is asked to lie upon the table and raise his torso backward in extension while his physician resists with a moderate degree of force the movement by placing his hands over the area wherein the lesion previously existed. Secondary extension lesions should be corrected if they remain after the adjustment of the primary lesions.

Unnecessary flexion movements on the part of the patient should be forbidden until the extensor muscles have gained strength and a power of contractility sufficient to prevent lesion under the influence of ordinary stress.

EXTENSION LESIONS

An extension lesion is a subluxation, or an immobilization, of a vertebral articulation in the position of extension. The inferior articular facets of the vertebra in lesion have glided downward upon the superior articular facets of the vertebra below usually to the point of interruption by the laminæ or until the spinous processes have come in contact and in this position immobilization has resulted from inflammatory changes.

From the study of the normal movement of extension, the anatomical relations present in extension may be deduced:

Spinous process.—Approximated to the one below, separated from the one above.

Body.—Slightly posterior at the anterior inferior margin.

Disc.—Compressed posteriorly and stretched somewhat anteriorly.

Ligaments

- I. Stretched, thinned, and atrophied
  - a. Anterior longitudinal.
- II. Relaxed and thickened, all posterior ligaments.

Intervertebral foramina.—Narrowed vertically with deposition of connective tissue lessening their calibre.

Muscles.—Fasciculi of the extensor muscles of that area contractured; corresponding flexor muscles stretched and atrophied.

Among the lumbar vertebræ the one most commonly in extension subluxation is the fifth; among the dorsals, any one from the third to the seventh. These lesions occur by groups also, the reason being faulty standing position due primarily to weakness from infectious illnesses, malnutrition, or hereditary tendencies; secondarily to traumatism, strain, fibrous ankylosis above or below; when extensive, they are characterized usually as the straight spine, and are caused by a posterior sacrum. When present in the cervical region, the cause may be a bilaterally posterior occiput or an upper dorsal kyphosis.

Extension lesions are less frequent, when primary, than flexion lesions, the reason doubtless being that they are less often produced by traumatism. The weight of the body carries the vertebræ into flexion more naturally than into extension, hence these lesions would be more common. Counterbalancing extension lesions are frequent, following the occurrence of a flexion lesion below.

Extension lesions are caused by traumatism; strain, usually from an attempt to regain equilibrium in falling; concussions; infections resulting in inflammation; muscular contraction, from irritation, and from the necessity of supporting weight anteriorly, as in obesity, pregnancy, abdominal tumors. In a patient having a barrel chest from emphysema often may be found a fifth lumbar extension lesion. From the weight of the shoulder girdle or an uncompensated posteriorly bilateral occipital lesion there may result an extension lesion of an upper dorsal vertebra. From the atrophy of intervertebral discs in the

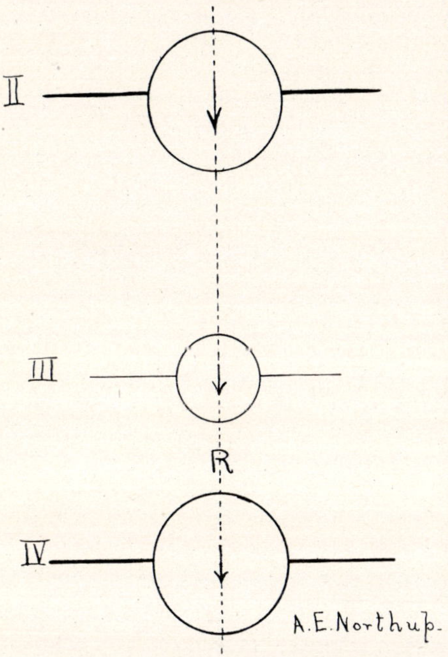

FIG. 31.—Schematic drawing to illustrate the approximation of the spinous process of the third thoracic with the fourth, in an extension lesion of the third-fourth joint. R, the interspace where restricted motion may be found. The smaller size of the circle, indicating the spinous process of the third, represents the flattening seen when looking at the line of spinous processes in the back.

aged, continued contraction of the lowest fasciculi of the multifidus spinæ and sacro-spinalis may result in an extension fifth lumbar lesion. High-heeled shoes may also be cited as a causal factor active in the same manner.

EXPERIMENTAL PALPATION, C.—Perform again experimental palpation, A.[1] If the fifth thoracic vertebra were immobilized in extension lesion, there would be no separation between its spinous process and that of the sixth; in forward flexion and in backward extension the approximation would remain unchanged. If the fifth were in extension lesion, its spine would be separated from the fourth above, but the distance between its spinous process and that of the fourth would be modified slightly by movement because the fourth-fifth articulation is assumed to be normal.

The diagnosis of an extension lesion may be stated in these terms:

THE SPINOUS PROCESS OF A VERTEBRA IN EXTENSION LESION IS APPROXIMATED TO THE SPINOUS PROCESS OF THE VERTEBRA BELOW AND MOVEMENT OF THAT AREA OF THE SPINE DOES NOT CHANGE THE RELATION OF THE SPINOUS PROCESSES.

EXPERIMENTAL PALPATION, D.—Perform again experimental palpation, B.[2] If the third lumbar vertebra were immobilized in extension lesion, there would be an approximation between its spinous process and that of the fourth and a separation between it and that of the second. Palpation would bring out the fact that motion is restricted in the interspace showing approximation of spinous processes. Although separation is apparent between the third and second, flexion and extension bring out evidence of normal movement in the articulation of the second-third lumbar joint.

Differential diagnosis will confirm preliminary diagnosis. An extension lesion of the third lumbar may be differentiated from

1. A second lumbar flexion lesion by the separation in the latter of the spinous process of the third from the second with restricted movement between the second and third and not between the third and fourth.

2. An anomalous condition in the third, a short spinous process, by the presence of unrestricted movement above and below the third lumbar in the latter condition.

3. A second lumbar showing the anomalous condition of a long spinous process by the detection of unrestricted motion in

1. See page 67, line 11.
2. See page 69, line 14.

the second-third lumbar joint and by the determination of the same amount of space between the spinous process of the second and those of the third and first. In the case of the lesioned vertebra there would be found restricted motion in the third-fourth lumbar joint.

4. An anomalous condition of the adjacent vertebræ, the third having a short spinous process, the fourth having a long spinous process. Absence of any restriction of movement in either the second-third or third-fourth spinal joints would confirm the diagnosis of irregular spinous processes.[1]

THE PRINCIPLE OF CORRECTION FOR EXTENSION LESIONS IS FLEXION.

GENERAL RULES.—THE ARTICULATING SURFACES MUST RETRACE THE PATH THEY TOOK IN THEIR DISPLACEMENT. The best leverage is obtained by means of pressure directed downward through the bodies of the vertebræ as low, perhaps, as the eighth thoracic or from below by flexion of the knees against the abdomen localizing as much as possible the force at the point of lesion by making the spinous process the fulcrum between the power arm and the weight arm. This method of correction is available in some patients as high as the tenth dorsal.

Correction of middorsal extension lesions or in fact of any of the dorsal extension lesions, is not without its difficulties, for these lesions afford less opportunity for direct leverage, and due to the thickening of relaxed ligaments and proliferation about the lesioned joint, the adjustment is often a problem deserving serious consideration. Preparatory treatment is usually required. It should be of such a nature that all ligaments shall receive physiological stimulation, by putting the joint through every possible movement, in particular the movements of rotation-sidebending and sidebending-rotation. For the upper five or six thoracics this is often best accomplished with the patient lying upon the side facing the physician, who carries the patient's head upon his forearm while his hand protects the neck and prevents a waste of force in rotation and sidebending in the cervical area; the thumb of the other hand is placed above each upper thoracic spinous

1. Extension lesions have been spoken of in the earlier literature of osteopathy as anterior spinal lesions for the reason that the spinous process by its approximation to the one below has appeared to be anterior in the line of spinous processes.

process in turn while the head is turned toward the upper shoulder preceded by a slight amount of face-turning. The thumb is then placed beneath the spinous process to pull it upward while the head is, after slight flexion, sidebent to the upper shoulder, face-turning to the table preceding the sidebending. After these two movements, attempted flexion and extension of the articulation should be made before an exact corrective movement is given.

CORRECTIVE MOVEMENTS

VIII. BEDSIDE MOVEMENT.—Let us assume an extension lesion of the second thoracic. B lies supine upon the table. O places one hand upon B's second ribs anteriorly, while the first finger of the other hand reaches underneath B's neck to exert a prying force upward on the spinous process of the second dorsal toward the head which rests upon O's forearm. The two hands work simultaneously.

This may be used with advantage in bedside treatment for any one of the four upper dorsals. It depends somewhat upon the tension that exists at the joint, whether a decided increase of force is required at the conclusion for adjustment.

IX. VERTEX PRESSURE MOVEMENT.—It is assumed that B has an extension lesion of the fifth dorsal. B sits upon the table, O standing behind him. B is directed to clasp his hands and place them upon the top of his head. O carries his arms under B's axillæ and reaching up grasps his wrists. He pulls straight downward to direct the line of force through the vertebral bodies and intervertebral discs. B is then carried forward and backward until by his muscle sense O ascertains at what angle he may best compress the fifth-sixth disc.[1] O may make posterior pressure against the angles of the ribs, as high as the fifth for the purpose of assisting to force the vertebra into flexion by the pull upon the transverse processes.[2] The pull downward upon the top of the head exerts a tremendous force and should be carefully used.

This corrective movement will adjust any midthoracic extension lesion.

1. One should always attempt to localize sharply any corrective movement.

2. The danger sometimes met with in a careless performance of this movement is that the osteopath may forget that flexion is the corrective principle and by carelessly swinging the patient backward, may cause a secondary extension lesion below or above.

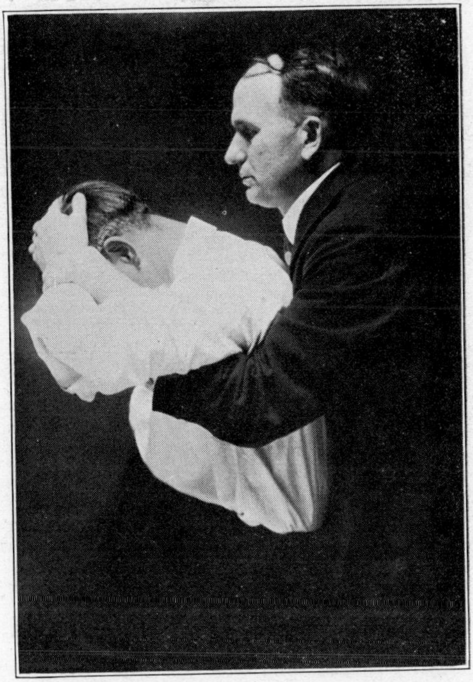

Fig. 32.—Illustrating the vertex pressure movement.

X. Spinous Fixed Point Movement.—It may be assumed that B has an extension lesion of the seventh thoracic. B sits upon a stool while O stands at his side. O places his thumb upon the spinous process of the eighth thoracic as a fixed point and maintains a firm pressure thereon. (This movement is illustrated by figure 26, page 68.) O places his other hand upon B's head to produce flexion of the upper thoracic area. He moves B's head forward in flexion until he finds the angle at which increased force may adjust the lesion. He then brings a force downward upon the top of B's head and through the vertebral bodies and discs until, by the opposition of the force directed against the fixed point, the two forces meet and the seventh-eighth articulation is adjusted. O may place his knee in the lumbar area of B's spine to hold that area in extension.

This movement may be used to adjust extension lesions of any of the thoracic vertebræ from the second to the ninth, inclusive.

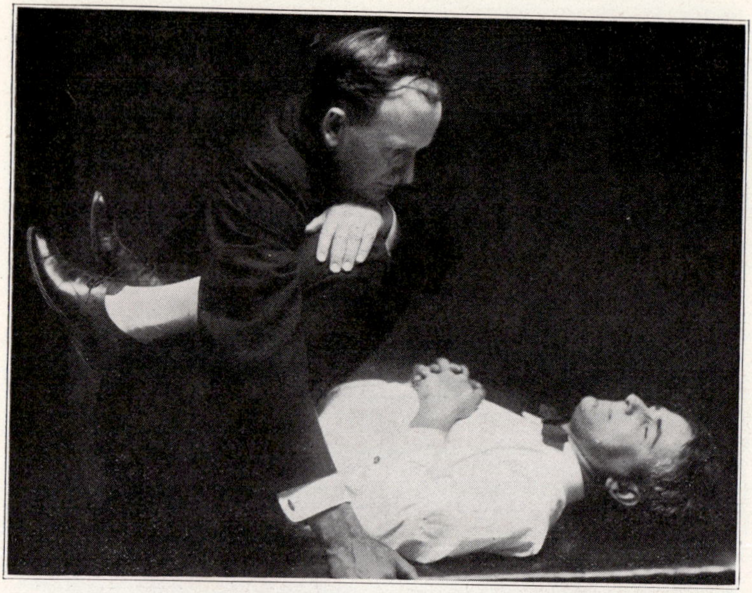

FIG. 33.—Illustrating the knee leverage movement.

XI. LONG LEVER MOVEMENT.—B is assumed to have an extension lesion of the eleventh thoracic. B sits upon the side of the table. O sits upon a high stool close to the table with his knees under the edge of the table by means of which he may brace himself in order to exert a strong pull downward. B clasps his hands easily upon the top or the back of his head. O passes his hands under B's axillæ and up over his chest grasping B's shoulders as near to the nape of his neck as possible.[1] B is then asked to flex his body forward while O tests the angle of forward flexion required to bring the force most directly downward through the vertebral bodies and the discs against the eleventh-twelfth disc which is stretched anteriorly. The adjustment is made by a strong pull downward.

XII. KNEE LEVERAGE MOVEMENT.—B is assumed to have an extension lesion of the fifth lumbar. He lies upon his back on a low table with his knees flexed against his abdomen. O places his chest against B's knees, his hands under B's spine to assist in guiding the direction of force. Sufficient pressure is brought

1. O's hands should be applied to the nape of B's neck rather than to the top of his head or to his neck, for the fault of the lever is its length, which for mechanical advantage should be shortened as much as possible.

against B's knees and through them transmitted to the contracted and shortened muscles and ligaments of the articulation in lesion, to effect a separation and adjust the lesion. B should then be turned upon his side with a firm hold upon the spinous process of the vertebra recently in subluxation, while extension is made of the joint above. The joint should then be put through sidebending-rotation, and the patient directed to practice flexion exercises for a few days, such as bending to touch the hands to the floor from the erect position, taking care not to pass the normal erect posture upon the return movement, nor to use the lower fasciculi of the sacro-spinalis and multifidus spinæ to pull himself up. A chair may be placed beside him which he may use to help regain the erect position.

XIII. FLOOR MOVEMENT.—The patient presents an extension lesion of the third lumbar. By reason of an ankylosed knee and corpulence, B cannot be treated by movement XII. B is asked to lie comfortably upon the floor. O grasps B's feet and carries

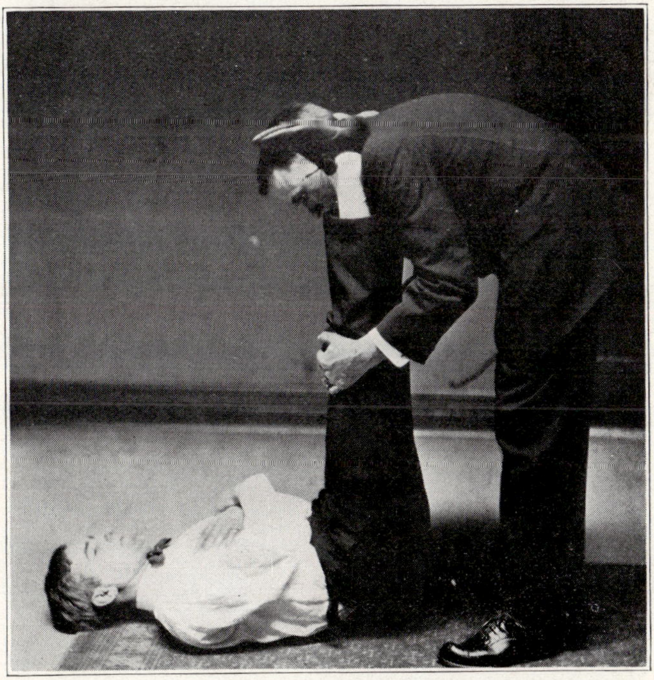

FIG. 34.—Illustrating the floor movement for an extension lesion of a lumbar vertebra.

them over his shoulder. He then steps between B's legs and bends forward taking hold of his thighs just above the knees. He raises B's hips and carries them back toward the floor a few times, until he has acquired a knowledge of the exact angle at which adjustment may be obtained. Pushing forward with the shoulders against B's heels, and pulling backward and thrusting downward upon B's thighs, a sudden increase of force is applied and the adjustment made.

Group lesions may be overcome by any method which has for its purpose the development of tone in stretched muscles, a stretching of contractured muscles, and the return to the normal of atonic ligaments. Flexion and extension with the patient lying upon the side is suggested for such patients. Forcible flexion of each joint in turn with the patient supine at the end of the table, knees flexed against the abdomen, and legs against the thighs is recommended. This last movement is the one which most quickly relieves the sacral pain, which is the common accompaniment of extension lesions of the lower lumbars, in fact it is palliative in cases of lumbago from uncorrected sidebending-rotation lesion of any lumbar vertebra.

CHAPTER V.

ROTATION AND SIDEBENDING LESIONS

ROTATION LESIONS

A rotation[1] lesion is a subluxation, or an immobilization, of a thoracic or cervical vertebral articulation in the position of rotation. In application of the above definition a third thoracic rotation lesion to the right may be defined as a lesion in which the third-fourth thoracic joint is immobilized in the position of rotation to the left.

In the normal movement of spinal rotation, it has been observed that the body of the vertebra rotates toward the side toward which torso rotation takes place; that, by the rotation of

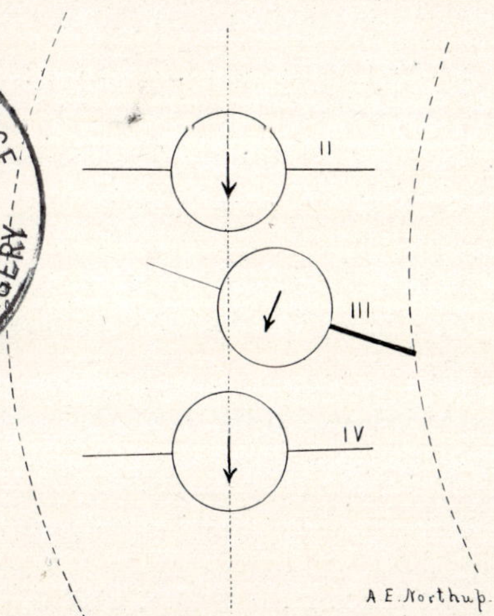

FIG. 35.—Schematic drawing to illustrate the rotation of the third thoracic vertebra in a left rotation lesion of the third-fourth thoracic joint. The arrows represent the direction toward which the spinous processes point. The circles, the bodies of the vertebræ. The horizontal lines, the transverse processes. The heavy line, the right transverse process approximated to that of the fourth and posterior. The light line, the left, separated from the fourth and anterior. The dotted lines, the concavity and convexity in the general movement of rotation to the right.

1. The whole term for the lesion should be rotation-sidebending, but for the purpose of simplifying the terminology, the second word has been discarded.

the whole vertebra, the spinous process turns to the opposite side; that each vertebra has tilted as a whole toward the side toward which it has rotated, and that the transverse process upon that side has moved backward and is also inclined sidewise because rotation in the spinal column is never a simple movement.[1]

If by reason of strain or any of the causes which are operative in the production of lesion, a thoracic vertebra should be immobilized in the position of rotation, the relation of the anatomical structures would be as follows, assuming that the third thoracic has been the one immobilized in rotation to the left:

1. Spinous process to the right.
2. Left transverse process posterior in relation to the second and fourth, approximated to the fourth, separated from the second.
3. Right transverse process slightly anterior in relation to adjacent transverse processes, separated from the fourth, approximated to the second.
4. Vertebral body rotated toward the left.
5. Intervertebral disc compressed upon the left and spread upon the right.
6. Perpendicular line projected upward from the superior surface of the vertebral body inclined to the left.
7. Intervertebral foramen on the left narrowed vertically, on the right widened vertically.
8. The third left rib slightly posterior to the adjacent ribs, approximated to the fourth, separated from the second.
9. The third right rib slightly anterior to adjacent ribs, separated from the fourth rib and approximated to the second rib.
10. Ligamentous changes.—On the left the anterior longitudinal, lateral spinal, capsular, and flava ligaments, in particular, are shortened and thickened; on the right the same ligaments are stretched, thinned, and atrophied.
11. Muscles.—Fasciculi of the multifidus, semispinalis, and the rotatores are contractured on the right, stretched and atrophied on the left.

EXPERIMENTAL PALPATION, E.—Ask the patient, B, who is assumed to have a rotation lesion of the third thoracic to the right,[2] to sit upon a stool in front of O, who inspects the upper part of

---

1. See page 22.

2. Rotation lesions are named according to the direction toward which the spinous process turns; thus, a rotation lesion of the third thoracic means that the spinous process is turned toward the right; the body of the vertebra, which of course may not be seen in inspection of the back, is turned to the left. The osteopathist has named the lesion from what he has seen.

his back. If B is not too well covered with adipose tissue, the spinous process of the third thoracic will be seen to be out of alinement with those above and below, being slightly to the right. It may be necessary to have B flex his head slightly and cross his arms easily in his lap to bring into view the deviation of the spinous process of the third. A deviation of the spinous process above, or of the one below, may be noted at the same time. B should be asked to turn his head to the right and then to the left. It will be noted that rotation to the left is much more easily accomplished.

O should place his finger-tips between the spinous processes of the third and fourth and of the second and third thoracic vertebræ. With his hand upon the top of B's head, O should produce the normal movements in B's spine, noting whether or not there are changes in the distance between the spinous processes. If there is restricted or lost motion in the third-fourth thoracic joint, there will be no change in the relation of the vertebræ upon movement. In the presence of lesion of the third only, movement should be present in the second-third joint.

For the palpation of the thoracic joints in normal rotation, the fingers should be placed along the lateral margins of the spinous processes for the purpose of comparing the movement of the spinous processes as the vertebræ rotate normally. When the head is turned to the left, it may be noted that the first thoracic spinous process turns to the right slightly beyond the second, the second beyond the third, and so on down the spinal column as far as rotation is the normal function of the spinal joints.

When a rotation lesion of the third thoracic is present, turning the head to the right or left does not cause the spinous process of the third to move laterally.

O should then palpate the intertransverse spaces to note whether or not the left third-fourth interspace is wider than the right; he should also palpate the left transverse process and the left third rib, both of which should be prominent posteriorly.

Counterbalancing lesions are usually present and they are of the same type as the primary lesion, that is, a rotation lesion to the right will induce a rotation lesion to the left in a vertebra above or below, most commonly in the vertebra immediately above. The induced or secondary lesion has for its purpose restoration of normal balance and therefore lacks many of the characteristics of the primary lesion. Its relations to the vertebra below are the same as regards osseous processes, but the soft tissues show no pathological effects. Contractions of muscles may be found but no contractures. If foramina are narrowed, the effects are minimum. Correction of the primary lesion is sufficient in ordinary cases for as soon as equilibrium is restored, secondary effects have no further reason to exist. A small amount of direct work will overcome them should they remain.

The diagnosis of the secondary lesion depends upon two things, the appearance when at rest of a lesion to the opposite side and the presence of unrestricted motion in the joint when subjected to experimental palpation.

Differential diagnosis is determined by the functional test of motion. A right rotation lesion of the third thoracic is to be differentiated from a deflected spinous process of the same vertebra by the presence of normal movement in the joint and by the absence of a counterbalancing lesion. Differentiation from a sidebending lesion will be considered later.[1]

Rotation subluxations occur as low as the tenth thoracic; below the tenth they are traumatic in character and the pathological changes in the articulation are greater, the symptoms more severe, and correction less easily accomplished. The causes operating to produce rotation lesions are those mentioned before.[2]

CORRECTIVE MOVEMENTS

THE PRINCIPLE OF CORRECTION FOR ROTATION LESIONS IS ROTATION TO THE OPPOSITE SIDE.

GENERAL RULES.—SINCE ROTATION IS ALWAYS ACCOMPANIED BY SIDEBENDING A ROTATION LESION MAY BE CORRECTED BY PLACING THE PATIENT IN THE POSITION OF ROTATION AND USING THE MOVEMENT OF SIDEBENDING FOR ADJUSTMENT.

Replacement of rotation lesions of the upper thoracic area should be made with the patient in the erect or moderately flexed position for the reason that rotation is normal to this area in either of these positions.

Rotation lesions of the eighth, ninth, and tenth thoracic vertebrae should be corrected with the patient erect.

Rotation lesions at the dorsolumbar junction, when not trau-

1. See page 105, the last line.
2. See page 10, paragraph 2. That which has been said concerning the gradual production of flexion lesions (page 71, line 20) might be applied to the production of other lesions.

matic lesions, are produced by strain with the patient in a position of hyperextension, therefore, hyperextension is the regular position for indicated corrective purposes.

Traumatic lesions[1] of the lumbar area may be corrected with the patient in the position of hyperextension; they are better adjusted by using the normal movement of that area, sidebending; they are most successfully overcome by the traction method[2] of correction.

I. HEAD-LEVERAGE MOVEMENT.—A patient, B, is assumed to have a right rotation lesion of the third thoracic vertebra. Ask B to lie upon his left side on the table. O stands beside the table facing him. O lifts B's head and rests it upon his right forearm, his hand encircling B's neck for the purpose of protecting the

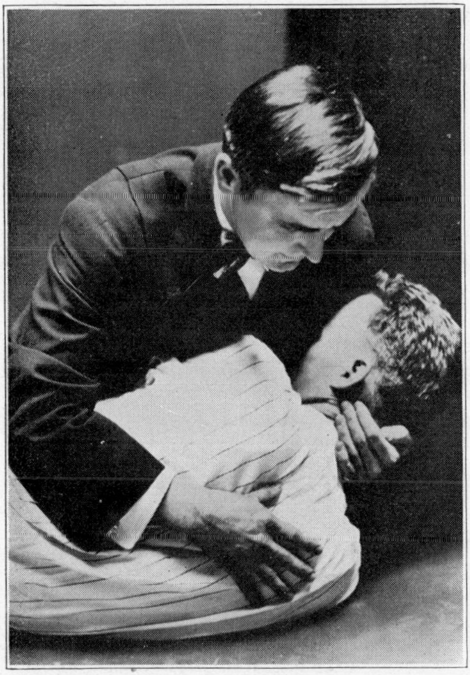

FIG. 36.—Illustrating the head-leverage movement for a left rotation lesion of the third thoracic vertebra.

1. See page 11, paragraph 5.
2. See page 72, paragraph 2.

cervical area against possible strain. O places the thumb of his left hand against the upper or right side of the spinous process of the vertebra in lesion.

O turns B's face toward the right in an arc of about thirty degress and then sidebends B's head to the right until the tension of the protective musculature is overcome. In securing this relaxation it may be necessary to make a few movements of flexion and extension among the movements aimed at correction. When relaxation is complete, O simultaneously exerts an additional amount of pressure against the spinous process and carries the head to the fullest extent of sidebending. It is common for the last movement to be finished with a slight popping sound, but it must not be supposed that this sound reports the adjustment of the lesion. It is probably the sound occasioned by the separation of articular facets. The adjustive movement must be continued beyond the moment of the popping noise.

Some assistance in localizing the movement to the upper thoracic area may be had by O's resting his chest against B's right shoulder and the lateral wall of his thorax, the pressure against his ribs holding the vertebræ below the one in lesion immobile.

II. SHOULDER-LIMITING MOVEMENT.—Let B sit upon the end of the table. O should stand to his left and slightly behind him. O places his left axilla over B's left shoulder, his forearm against the side of B's head, his hand on the top of B's head. O places his right thumb against the right side of the third thoracic spinous process and exerts pressure in an effort to move it to the left and turn the body of the vertebra from the left toward the right. At the same time O turns B's head toward the right slightly and then sidebends the head to the same side, performing a series of sidebending movements to secure relaxation. O maintains a firm pressure downward upon B's shoulder to limit the area of sidebending to that controlled by the leverage of head and neck. When relaxation is complete, a slight increase of pressure against the point of attack, the spinous process, and an added impetus to sidebending will adjust the lesion. If the popping sound should be heard, sidebending must be carried a degree further.

The movements above will adjust any rotation lesion of the upper four thoracic vertebræ.

III. RIB-LEVERAGE MOVEMENT.—Let B sit upon a stool. O stands to the right and in front of B. He places his right arm under B's left axilla and rests his middle finger upon B's left third rib, the one which is prominent posteriorly in a right rotation lesion of the third thoracic vertebra. O's left thumb should be placed against the right side of the spinous process of the third in the effort to turn it toward the left. By pulling with his right arm or by pressing against B's right shoulder with his shoulder, O turns B toward the right in simple rotation. When relaxation has been secured, adjustment is made by a slight increase in rotation and an additional amount of pressure against the angle of the third rib. B may rest his head against O's chest in ease, turning his face to the right when the lesion is a right rotation lesion.

The minutiæ of the above movement may be changed to suit the case. In large patients, O's left hand may be placed against B's right shoulder to make the rotation more forceful. B should be turned as far to the right as possible and at the moment of adjustment turned still farther.[1] O may place the forefinger of his left hand against the left side of the spinous process of B's fourth thoracic vertebra, to make a fixed point against which to rotate the area above.

This movement may be used to adjust rotation lesions of the thoracic vertebræ from the third to the eighth inclusive.

IV. FORWARD-BENDING MOVEMENT.—B is assumed to have a right rotation lesion of the eighth thoracic vertebra. Let B sit upon a stool, while O stands to his right and bends forward until his back is level with B's right axilla. B is asked to turn very slightly and place both arms across O's back. O places his right arm across B's chest, under his left axilla, his hand over B's left ribs from the sixth to the ninth. O's left thumb pushes against the spinous process of the eighth thoracic for the purpose of turning the vertebra from the left toward the right. Simultaneously O rotates B's body to the right by pulling with his right hand and swinging his own bdy forward.

Several movements are made, aimed at correction. When relaxation has been obtained, rotation is carried as far as possible and completed with an extra forcible movement, which should adjust the lesion if both hands work in unison and the action is rightly timed.

The movement may be varied by having O put the corrective pressure against the prominent eighth left rib, while with his left hand he grasps B's right wrist and by swinging his weight forward rotates B's body farther to the right and then finishes the movement

1. There is a certain knack in knowing when the tension of muscles has been released sufficiently to warrant an attempt at adjustment This is acquired after many months of practice and it is the result of the cultivation of the sensations coming from muscles, tendons, and joints.

2. It is held by many osteopathists that adjustment is made of the whole area above, including the vertebra in lesion, to the vertebra below. In the case cited, the spine from the third dorsal up would be considered adjusted to the fourth dorsal when the third-fourth joint became normalized.

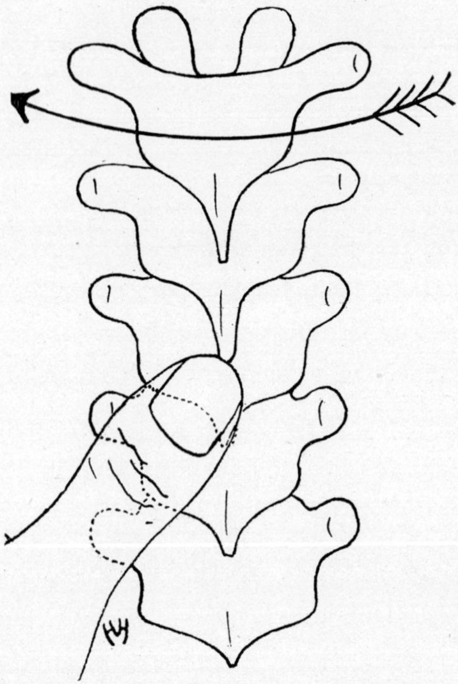

FIG. 37.—Illustrating the pressure of the thumb against the spinous process in the correction of a rotation lesion of the tenth dorsal to the left. The arrow points to the side toward which the rotation of the body for correction should be made.

with secondary sidebending which adds compression on the right to the intervertebral disc between the eighth and ninth thoracic vertebræ, gaps the articulation on the left and causes the left side of the disc to rebound.

This movement will adjust rotation lesions from the sixth to tenth thoracic inclusive.

V. HALF-LEANING MOVEMENT.—B is assumed to have a right rotation lesion of the fifth thoracic vertebra. Let B sit well back upon a stool, behind which O sits on a table. O leans slightly forward and B rests comfortably backward against O's right shoulder. O places the thumb of his left hand against the angle of the fifth left rib or against the left transverse process of the fifth thoracic vertebra. O places his right arm around B, under his right axilla and forward until he lays his hand over the anterior extremity of the left fifth rib. O rotates B's torso slightly, lifting a little on the fifth rib from both extremities. When relaxation is felt to be complete, a sudden increase of rotation and of pressure against the posterior extremity of the fifth rib will adjust the lesion.

This corrective movement is suitable for the adjustment of rotation lesions of the fifth to ninth thoracic vertebræ inclusive.

VI. TRACTION SIDEBENDING MOVEMENT.—B is assumed to have a right rotation lesion of the tenth thoracic. B sits upon a low stool. O stands in front of B and to the left. He places his left knee inside of B's knees to assist in making immobile B's pelvis. O reaches around B with both arms, under B's axillæ, and, if B is not too large, he grasps the spinous process of the eleventh thoracic vertebra from the left side to make of it a fixed point. With his right hand he takes a firm hold upon the upper part of B's spine or under his left scapula, or he may grasp the spinous process of the vertebra in lesion to pull it toward the left. O then swings B in gentle rotation to the right, lifts B with slight traction, and as soon as he feels resistance is overcome, he sidebends B to the right. The secondary sidebending with the holding of the vertebra below immovable should not fail to adjust any rotation lesion of a lower thoracic vertebra. If the rotation lesion is of the last two thoracics or upper two lumbars, B may be carried back in some hyperextension before the rotation is begun and the hyperextension must be maintained through the movement.

VII. HOOP-ROLLING MOVEMENT.—B is assumed to have the same lesion as in the last instance. He lies upon his left side upon the table. O stands in front of him, and places his right hand against B's right shoulder or in his right axilla. O directs B to place his left leg behind the right on the able and bend the right leg at the knee. O puts his left forearm on B's right hip, a finger against the left side of the eleventh thoracic spinous process to make of it a fixed point. O rotates B's torso to the right by pushing his right shoulder backward. He may need to repeat the operation several times until resistance has been overcome, when by a sudden increase of rotation the tenth thoracic returns to normal alinement with the eleventh.

AFTER-TREATMENT

Rotation lesions that may be said to be in the chronic stage, are often exceedingly difficult to adjust; they require time and patience on the part both of physician and patient, skill to accomplish the correction, and care to avoid a recurrence of the deviation from the normal alinement. Atrophic muscles must be stimulated to recovery; to that end patients must be advised to take exercises which will bring tone to these muscles, the best of which would be strong rotation to the side of the spinous process. Since the patient knows practically nothing of the condition of his or her spine, he or she must be told to which side to turn the head and body. If the lesion is the common rotation lesion of the second thoracic, an excellent exercise which localizes the action almost directly at the joint in lesion is first, extreme flexion of the head and upper part of the body, then turning the head as far as possible to the side of the spinous process. It has been pointed out that in extreme flexion rotation is limited to the last two cervical and upper two thoracic vertebræ.[1]

Muscles that were contractured must be given no opportunity to contract strongly; for that reason it is often required of the physician to enumerate the actions that tend to reproduce the lesion, as, upward reaching with the arms, often followed by a lowering of heavy objects which necessitates a turning of the head to get it out of the way, or unusually strong action of one arm; the habit of turning the head toward objects which have been put in a certain place that for the individual is harmful, as, a clock, an outside window, a chart, a mirror, a book of reference; the knee-chest position with the head not turned to the side of the spinous process; sleeping on the chest with the face turned to the side; sleeping on the side with a pillow that is too high so that the head is sidebent in the position of rest; napping in a chair with the head dropping over the shoulder. In the case of lower dorsal lesions, heavy lifting with one arm is the most frequent cause of the recurrence of the lesion. Students having rotation lesions should be especially careful about their sitting positions in studying and writing.

LATERAL LUMBAR LESIONS

When the spinous process of a lumbar vertebra is out of alinement with its fellows, it may be assumed to be in lateral lesion. According to the movements that are possible to that area under the stress of force, there may be two kinds of lateral lumbar lesions:

1. See page 25, line 17.

I. A subluxation, an immobilization of a lumbar vertebral articulation in the position of sidebending.

II. A traumatic lesion, an immobilization of a lumbar vertebral articulation in the position of rotation.[1]

It has been proved by experiment,[2] that the bodies of the lumbar vertebræ turn to the concavity of the curve in sidebending. Since in rotation in the cervical and thoracic areas the vertebral bodies turn to the concavity of the curve, the same holds true of the traumatic lesions of the lumbar area. If in both lesions the bodies of the vertebræ turn to the same side, the anatomical relations of the vertebra in lesion are practically the same as in a thoracic rotation lesion,[3] aside from the relation of the planes of the articulating surfaces,[4] the pathological effects in ligaments and surrounding tissues,[5] and the obvious fact that in rotation a vertebra turns in a larger arc than in sidebending-rotation, wherein rotation is secondary; hence the lumbar spinous process is not deviated from the median line as far as the thoracic spinous process in a rotation lesion.

EXPERIMENTAL PALPATION, E.—B is assumed to have a right lateral lesion of the third lumbar vertebra. He is asked to sit erect upon the end of the table. O standing behind him observes that the spinous process of the third is lateral to the right in comparison with the contiguous spinous processes. If his muscular tissues are so thick that the line of processes may not be easily seen, he may be asked to bend forward in moderate flexion. The spinous process of the second or the first may be found lateral to the left. B is asked to bend sidewise to the right and to the left. It may be observed that lateral flexion is more easily accomplished to the left than to the right.

---

1. See page 11, paragraph 5.
2. See experiment VI, page 28; also figure 7, page 27.
3. See page 88, paragraph 2.
4. See page 15, figure I. Since rotation is not normal to the lumbar area, save in cases having an anomalous fifth, the inferior articular facets of which face less medially and more backward, rotation would jam the planes of the articular surfaces. Dr. Kendall L. Achorn of Boston has brought to my attention several sacra in which the superior articular facets show wide deviations from the lumbar type. In the individual whose facets are like those of the thoracic articulations, only reverse in direction, rotation in the lumbosacral joint would be normal. In traumatic lesions of this area, the spinous process of the lesioned vertebra is usually found approximated to the one below, separated from the one above.
5. Necessarily greater in traumatic lesions due to the secondary effects of the violent wedging of the vertebra by a force applied in a direction physiologically abnormal to the joint.

O stands to the left and slightly in front of B, places his left hand on top of B's right shoulder, his right hand against the left side of the row of lumbar spinous processes to palpate the changes that may take place upon movement in that area. O now bends B sidewise to the right by pulling downward upon his right shoulder. At the same time he observes that the first lumbar spinous process moves to the left of the second, the second to the left of the third; the third remains stationary in regard to the fourth and they together move to the left of the fifth.

By moving his left hand to a place behind B's right scapula, it will be possible to bend B forward in flexion, and then by pushing with his left shoulder against B's chest O may carry him backward in extension. By palpating with the forefinger of the right hand between the spinous processes of the third and fourth, O may find that no motion in the third-fourth joint is manifest.

By reversing his position to the right and front of B, and placing his right hand upon B's left shoulder, he may bend him in left lateral flexion. It will be observed that the lumbar spinous processes, each in turn, move to the left of the one below except the third which remains immovable in relation to the fourth.

EXPERIMENTAL PALPATION, F.—Let B lie upon his left side upon the table, O standing beside the table facing him. O asks B to place the left leg, the one underneath, backward upon the table. He asks him to flex his right knee and place the right leg in advance of the left. A partial concavity then appears uppermost at B's waistline. To complete the position of sidebending, O may place beneath B's left shoulder a large, hard pillow, or the thickness of his forearm beneath the upper part of B's thorax. Since lateral lumbar lesions are produced usually by strain in sidebending-rotation, the movement may be accomplished with sidebending by position and rotation by movement.

B is then asked to place his right arm over O's right shoulder, while O places his right shoulder against the forward part of B's right shoulder or in his axilla. O places the finger of his left hand against the under side of the lumbar spinous processes to palpate for motion in those articulations. By pressing against B's shoulder, O may rotate B's trunk backward toward the right. It will be found that each spinous process in turn moves slightly to the left of the one below, until the third is reached, when it, being in lateral lesion upon the fourth, does not move except as the fourth moves, as one vertebra instead of two, to the left of the fifth spinous process.

In some people, who are more flexible than others, sidebending is possible as high as the eighth or ninth dorsal, and in the detection of lesion, this palpation may be used for lower thoracic lesions.

Particular attention should be paid to the second-third articulation when the spinous process of the second has appeared to be to the left of the median line of the back, for there is present with rare exception a secondary lesion of a vertebra above and that lesion has the characteristic that distinguishes it from a primary lesion, normal movement.

Lateral lumbar lesions are commonly the result of strain[1] in a return to the upright position after lateral or forward flexion, as in the lifting of heavy objects. Other strains are the lifting of large or heavy objects above the head, the effort in falling to save oneself, and the carrying of heavy weights at the side. The causes that have been mentioned, irritation causing muscular contraction, trauma, and infection, produce lumbar lesions with great frequency.

The most common cause for lumbago is a lateral lumbar lesion.[2] The patient gives the history of having stooped to pick up something and in rising of having been seized with a sudden pain in his back with inability to move. Careful questioning will elicit the fact that the movement was one of sidebending.

CORRECTIVE MOVEMENTS

THE PRINCIPLE OF CORRECTION FOR LATERAL LUMBAR LESIONS IS SIDEBENDING-ROTATION.

GENERAL RULES.—SINCE SIDEBENDING IS ALWAYS ACCOMPANIED BY ROTATION A LATERAL LUMBAR LESION MAY BE CORRECTED BY PLACING THE PATIENT IN THE POSITION OF SIDEBENDING AND USING THE MOVEMENT OF ROTATION FOR ADJUSTMENT.

Lumbar sidebending is normal alike in the erect and hyperextended positions, therefore, lateral lumbar lesions may be corrected with the patient in the position of hyperextension.

---

1. It should not be forgotten that the lumbar area supports the body above and that the influence of the weight would be felt to a greater degree upon slight strain among the lumbars than elsewhere in the spine.

2. Lateral lumbar lesions are also etiologic in causing constipation of the large intestine, pelvic diseases, pain in the knee not caused by local pathology, weak ankles, and reflex conditions primarily induced by lumbar lesions. See Marion E. Clark's "Applied Anatomy," pages 241-296, published by the Journal Printing Co., Kirksville, Mo., 1906.

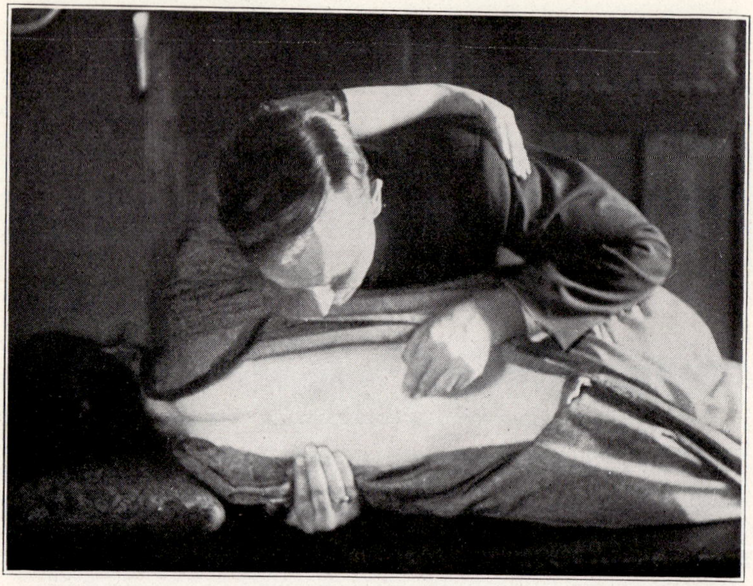

FIG. 38.—Illustrating the sidebending rolling movement for the correction of a right lateral lumbar lesion.

It is well to have in mind the compression of the disc on the side toward which the vertebral body has rotated so that in correction one may seek to stretch that side of the disc and compress the side that was widened by the sidetilting of the vertebra.[1]

VIII. SIDEBEND ROLLING MOVEMENT.—Let B be assumed to have a right lateral third lumbar lesion. He is placed upon the table in the position described in experimental palpation, F.[2] O places the elbow of his left arm strongly against B's right hip, a finger of the left hand underneath, to the left of, the spinous process of the fourth lumbar vertebra to make of it a fixed point. O may place the tip of another finger between the spinous processes of the fourth and fifth, on the left side of these processes, for the purpose of determining when the rotation that is given by pushing against B's right shoulder is sufficient to bring the force of secondary rotation to the third-fourth articulation. By this means the osteopathist may often get an idea of how much of a certain

1. The structural relations must be kept vividly in mind while execution is planned. There should be no uncertain manipulation of soft tissues or attempt at motion without a definite action in mind.

2. See page 98, paragraph 4.

movement is required to bring definite action upon an articulation. O then rotates B backward, toward B's right, until he knows that relaxation has been secured about the joint needing adjustment, when with a slight additional force in rotation and in making more fixed the fulcrum below, correction is accomplished. It is common to hear the popping sound in the correction of these lesions but it should be remembered that the movement falls short of adjustment unless it is continued a step beyond the amount of correction secured at the moment the popping report is made.[1]

This movement will adjust lateral lesions of any vertebra from the ninth thoracic to the fifth lumbar inclusive. In the lower thoracic region sidebending occurs more often than rotation in the movement of that area of the spine.

IX. HYPEREXTENSION SIDEBENDING MOVEMENT.—Let B, having the same lesion as above, sit upon a stool of moderate height. O stands in front of him and to his left. O reaches around B to take a firm hold of his trunk so that he may carry him back in slight hyperextension. He makes the necessary sidebending to the right, which by position is essential to correction; he then follows sidebending with rotation to the right. Traction is often used with this movement and precedes sidebending. Experience in the sensations from muscles, tendons, and joints, is necessary to the successful use of this movement for adjustment of a particular lesion for, with the arms about the patient lifting him, there is no opportunity to employ a fixed point and in consequence of this lack of localization, there may be indiscriminate movement of lumbar joints with many popping sounds and without securing adjustment of the third-fourth lesion.

X. KNEE-BENDING MOVEMENT.—B is assumed to have a right lateral lesion of the fifth lumbar vertebra. He is asked to sit upon a stool of moderate height, while O kneels upon his right knee to the right of B. O passes his right arm across B's chest under his left arm and lays his hand over B's left ribs. Reaching across B's back, he grasps the anterior superior spine of B's left innominate to hold the pelvis immobile. O asks B to bend his body sidewise over O's back and lay his arms outstretched in advance of his body. By pulling with his right arm and holding the pelvis fixed with his left, O rotates B's torso to the right, in secondary rotation, several times in gradually increasing arcs until

1. It is regrettable that so many osteopathists have not followed more closely the many experiments of Dr. Carl McConnell so that the popping sound and its secondary effects are well understood. The reader is urged to read Dr. McConnell's own words upon this subject, in the Journal of the A. O. A., May, 1913, page 547.

he is conscious that B understands the direction of the movement and has relaxed sufficiently to make adjustment possible by further increase of rotation.

One may by placing the finger or thumb against the left side of any lumbar vertebra, make a fixed point against which one may adjust a sidebending lesion of the vertebra above.

AFTER-TREATMENT

Since the mass of muscles in the lumbar area is the largest of the back, it is essential that, after the unbalance resulting upon lesion, effort should be made to secure a restoration to normal action in these muscles; for this reason movements that will exercise both groups equally[1] should be taken for some time and the patient not dismissed until the physician has noted a return to power of all the atonic fasciculi.

All movements that tend toward sidebending to the side opposite the former position of the spinous process should be avoided; leaning to the same side, taken as a conscious effort and with some resistance, will hasten the process of muscle building. Upward reaching with the hand upon that side must be avoided also, for a concavity to the opposite side would be produced and a possible recurrence of the lesion follow.

At each treatment the joint should be put through its normal movements as far as possible and especially following correction for the reason that ligamentous tissues are directly acted upon in this way. Preceding correction, flexion and extension will often help to secure the relaxation so often helpful to a ready adjustment of the lesion.

SIDEBENDING LESIONS

When sidebending is normal to the thoracic area, it has been demonstrated,[2] it follows forward flexion and the bodies of the vertebræ rotate to the convexity of the curve. According to the definition[3] of a subluxation, a sidebending lesion of a thoracic

1. For example, backward bending, forward flexion, and upward reaching with both arms.

2. See page 28, experiment IX.

3. See page 11, line 17.

vertebra may be defined as an immobilization of that vertebra in the position of primary forward bending and secondary lateral flexion. When a superior sidebending force is directed against an almost defenseless articulation in the position of erectness or hyperextension, a lateral lesion of that vertebra may result and from the character of its production it may be classified as a traumatic lesion.

It is altogether due to the character of the intervertebral disc that in sidebending-rotation the bodies of the vertebræ rotate

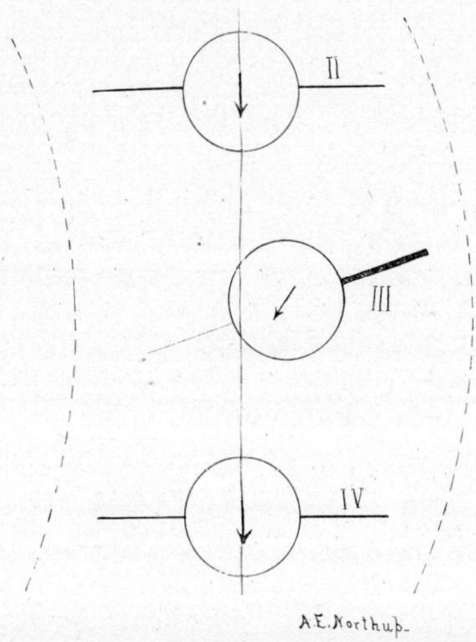

FIG. 39.—Schematic drawing to illustrate a sidebending lesion of the third thoracic to the left. The arrows indicate the direction in which the spinous process points. The heavy line, the right prominent transverse process. The light line, the slightly anterior transverse process of the third. The horizontal lines, the transverse processes of the second and fourth. The vertical line, the median line of vertebral bodies. The curved lines, the concavity and convexity of the original curve produced by sidebending to the left.

away from the side to which bending takes place. As has been explained in the discussion of the general movement of sidebending,[1] the intervertebral disc has already been compressed anteriorly; when sidebending follows, there is but one direction in which rotation of the vertebra is possible and that is away from further compression. The character of the disc is responsible for the same rotation in a traumatic lesion. Substances that are highly

1. See page 29, paragraphs one and three.

elastic rotate their mass and adjoining movable structures away from the constricting force in the pathway of least resistance.

These lesions are ordinarily produced as the result of strain in the position of forward flexion with sidebending in the effort to pick up a heavy object; in dodging a missile with a concluding sharp movement laterally, or by direct injury; more rarely by the other causes operative in the production of most lesions.

These lesions are spoken of as lateral thoracic lesions, in contra-distinction to the rotation lesions of the same area. They are named according to the direction toward which the spinous process points. A left lateral third thoracic would be named from the spinous process of the third being to the right of the median line of spinous processes. The anatomical relations of such a lesion would be as follows:

1. Spinous process of the third lateral to the left.

2. Vertebral body rotated to the right.

3. The right transverse process more prominent posteriorly than the adjacent transverse processes, separated from the fourth and approximated to the second.

4. The left transverse process less prominent than the adjoining transverse processes, approximated to the fourth and separated from the second.

6. The intervertebral disc compressed upon the left, widened upon the right.

6. The right third rib slightly posterior to adjacent ribs, separated from the fourth and approximated to the second.

7. The left third rib slightly anterior to adjacent ribs, approximated to the fourth and separated from the second.

8. A perpendicular line projected upward from the superior surface of the vertebral body, inclined to the left.

9. Intervertebral foramen on the left narrowed antero-posteriorly, on the right widened vertically.

10. Ligamentous changes.—On the right the anterior longitudinal, lateral spinal, capsular, and flava ligaments are stretched and atrophied; on the left the same ligaments are shortened and thickened.

11. Fasciculi of the multifidus and rotatores are stretched and atrophied on the right; fasciculi of the same muscles shortened and thickened on the left.

EXPERIMENTAL PALPATION, G.—Let the patient, B, sit upon a stool of moderate height, with the back exposed to inspection. If he has a lateral lesion of the third thoracic vertebra, the spinous process of that vertebra will be found to be slightly out of alinement with the ones above and below, not markedly deviated to the side but sufficiently out of alinement to be noted upon close inspection. B is asked to bend forward in slight flexion and then to sidebend his head and shoulders to the right and to the left. If the lesion is a right lateral third thoracic, it will be found that sidebending is more easily accomplished to the right than to the left for the reason that in sidebending the bodies of the vertebræ rotate to the convexity of the curve, hence bending away from the convexity is always much more easily done.

O should now place his finger-tips between the spinous processes of the third and fourth and the second and third for the purpose of palpating for mobility in those articulations. The patient's head should be moved backward and forward in flexion and extension. If lesion is present, there will be restricted motion between the spinous processes of the third and fourth vertebræ. The finger-tips should then be placed to the right of the spinous processes of the second, third, and fourth thoracic vertebræ to detect movement of these in sidebending to the right. If lesion is present in the third-fourth articulation, there will be no change in the relative positions of these upon movement. Sidebending to the left should elicit the same results. If secondary lesion above or below should be present, it would show practically no disturbance in motion.[1] These lesions will be of the same type as the primary lesion, thus, a primary sidebending lesion will induce a secondary sidebending lesion.[2]

Differential diagnosis must be made from a rotation lesion of the same vertebra and is made with great difficulty in persons who are obese or well covered with heavy spinal musculature. The objective signs are alike in that there is a deviation of the spinous process to the right, let us say, of the median line. The deviation is usually less in a lateral lesion than in a rotation lesion. By three means may we differentiate:

I. History.—The patient may be able to recall the time of the production of the lesion. If it was the result of a sidebending force of great intensity, unquestionably the lateral lesion is a traumatic one. If it was produced by sidebending in the position of forward flexion, the diagnosis should be considered as established in the absence of more pronounced signs.

2. Palpation.—In a right rotation lesion, the prominent left

---

1. See page 17, line 35, also page 18, line 1.
2. Cf. page 89, line paragraph 5.

third transverse process and the corresponding rib are approximated to the fourth and separated from the second.[1]

In a right sidebending lesion, the prominent left third transverse process and corresponding rib are separated from the fourth and approximated to the second.[2]

3. Therapeutic measures.—When following preliminary means of securing relaxation, the proper adjustive method of correction is applied for a rotation lesion and it fails to overcome the lesion, the corrective movements for a lateral third dorsal may be attempted with judgment and carefulness.[3]

A lateral lesion may need to be differentiated from a spinal anomaly, a vertebra having a deflected spinous process. In the latter case, motion will be found to be present in the articulations of which that vertebra forms a part. In the case of a lateral lesion to the right with a spinous process deflected to the left and in line or out of line with adjoining vertebral spinous processes, by the means mentioned above may diagnosis be determined. Such cases are the most difficult ones to diagnose and may need the skill of an experienced osteopathist.[4]

CORRECTIVE MOVEMENTS

THE PRINCIPLE OF CORRECTION FOR LATERAL THORACIC LESIONS IS SIDEBENDING IN FORWARD FLEXION TO THE SIDE OPPOSITE THE LESION.

GENERAL RULES.—SINCE SIDEBENDING IS A PART OF THE COMPOUND MOVEMENT OF SIDEBENDING-ROTATION, LATERAL THORACIC LESIONS MAY BE CORRECTED BY PLACING THE PATIENT IN

1. Reversing experiment I, page 23, when the subject, B, is rotated to the left, a curvature will be seen in his thoracic spinal area with the convexity to the right, the high side upon the left; therefore, in a single lesion, e. g., a right rotation lesion of the third, the left side will be the counterpart of the concavity of the original curve in the production of the lesion.

2. Experiment IX, page 28, presents the fact that when the spinous process points toward the concavity of the curve, the body of the vertebra has rotated toward the left, the convexity of the curve. The transverse process on that side would, naturally, be separated from its fellow below. See page 29, paragraph 1.

3. Palpation is the preferred method of differentiation. It is rare that by the histories of these cases can their diagnoses be made. The objection to the third means is that it has its dangers in the hands of any but watchful physicians.

4. Dr. C. P. McConnell, in the Journal of the A. O. A., Feb. 1913, page 355, pertinently remarks that the biggest problem in technique is careful diagnosis. The entire article should be read.

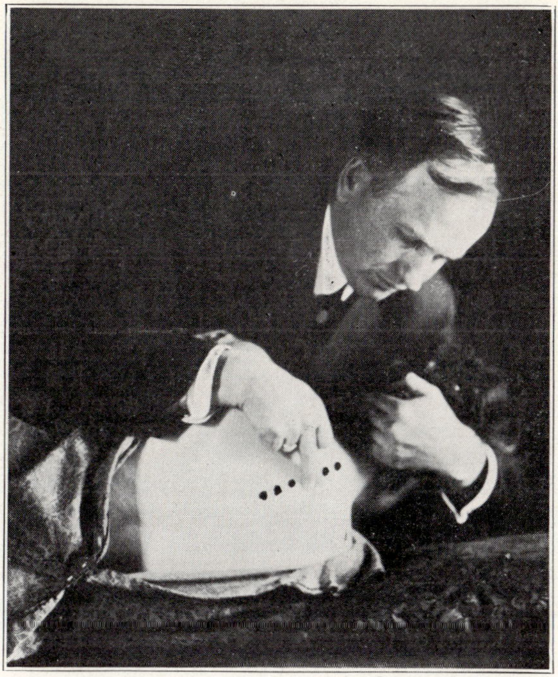

FIG. 40.—Illustrating the head-bending movement for the correction of a right lateral third dorsal lesion.

THE POSITION OF FLEXION-SIDEBENDING AND USING THE MOVEMENT OF ROTATION FOR ADJUSTMENT.

XI. HEAD-BENDING MOVEMENT.—B is assumed to have a right lateral lesion of the third thoracic. B is asked to lie upon his right side on the table. O places his left forearm under B's head, his hand encircling B's neck. He places the thumb, a finger, or a knuckle, underneath, to the right side of, the spinous process of the third to pull it toward the left. B's head is carried forward in slight flexion, his face turned to the right.[1] O then sidebends

1. The purpose of the turning of the face is to distinguish this movement from the head-leverage movement, I, page 91. The students have a memory scheme for the correcting of these lesions which reads, "In rotation lesions, turn the face and bend the head to the same side as the spinous process; in sidebending lesions, turn the face toward the spinous process and bend the head to the opposite side."

Turning the face toward the spinous process at least turns the bodies of the cervical vertebræ above in the direction it is desired to turn the body of the vertebra in lesion. I am not persuaded that it is of particular mechanical value unless the lesion be of the first thoracic.

B's head to the left, at the same time bringing stress against the spinous process in the effort to turn the vertebral body from the left toward the right. When relaxation has been secured, an increase of force will usually adjust the lesion. If the popping sound is heard, the sidebending must be carried slightly further.

XII. STOOL-AND-ARM MOVEMENT.—Let B, who is assumed to have the same lesion as in movement XI, sit upon the table, O standing upon his right side. O places his right axilla over B's right shoulder, his forearm along the side of B's head, his right hand on the top of B's head. He bends B's head in slight forward flexion, and then turns it toward the right, and sidebends it slightly to the left. He places the thumb of his left hand against the right side of the spinous process of the third and pushes it toward the left at the same time bending B's head to the left in greater lateral flexion. He repeats this movement several times. The moment B becomes accustomed to the movement of sidebending so that he relaxes perfectly, both pressure against the spinous process and sidebending should be increased until correction is made.

The last two movements will correct lateral lesions of the upper thoracic vertebræ from the first to the fourth inclusive.

XIII. LOCKED-ARMS MOVEMENT.—B is assumed to have a right lateral lesion of the seventh thoracic. He is asked to sit upon a stool of moderate height, to fold his arms in front of his chest, and to rest his head upon his arms, with his face turned to the right. O places his axilla over B's left shoulder, passes his left arm under B's folded arms and grasps B's right upper arm. B is carried forward in some flexion, O bending his knees if necessary to bring his chest to the level of B's head. O places his right thumb against the left side of the spinous process of the eighth thoracic vertebra to make a fixed point against which to sidebend B's seventh thoracic vertebra. O then sidebends B to the left strongly, and repeats the movement until B relaxes, upon which, with an increase of both pressure and sidebending, he is able to adjust the lateral seventh vertebra.

This movement may be varied by O's placing his thumb against the right side of the spinous process of the seventh to add rotation to sidebending of the vertebra in lesion. This may be changed by having O stand on the right of B and reverse his hands.

The above movement will adjust lateral thoracic lesions from the fifth to the eighth inclusive.

XIV. SHOULDER-DOWNWARD MOVEMENT.—Let B, who is assumed to have a right lateral ninth thoracic lesion, sit upon a stool, with O standing beside him to the right. O reaches across B's chest and grasps his left shoulder, at the same time placing the thumb of his left hand against the left side of the spinous process of the tenth thoracic to make of it a fixed point. O then bends B forward in slight flexion and then to the left, and repeats the lateral flexion until B is felt to relax, when O concludes the movement of lateral flexion with a slight amount of rotation to the left with increased reinforcement of the fixed point. Adjustment should then occur.

XV. SHOULDER-RAISING MOVEMENT.—Let B sit upon the table, with his feet resting upon a stool so that he will relax without a fear of falling. With a right lateral lesion of the ninth thoracic, O should stand to B's right, his right shoulder in B's right axilla. O should pass his right arm across B's chest, under his left axilla, with his hand resting upon the left ninth rib at the angle. B bends forward in very slight flexion. O places the thumb of his left hand against the right side of the spinous process of the ninth and pushes toward the left, at the same time raising B's right shoulder and sidebending B to the left, concluding the sidebending with secondary rotation. At the moment of relaxation, increase of pressure upon the left rib, against the spinous process, and sidebending-rotation to the left will serve to adjust the lesion.

The last two movements will correct lateral lesions of the thoracic vertebræ from the sixth to the ninth inclusive.

AFTER-TREATMENT

Resistance exercises[1] are of the utmost importance in the maintenance of the normalization of a joint that has been in sidebending lesion. For those patients who have had lateral lesions of the upper thoracic vertebræ, the resistance exercises must be taken in the position of extreme forward flexion for in this way there is a natural limitation placed upon the extent of the sidebending, localizing it to the area desired. Care must be taken in advising all exercises that the patient shall have no opportunity to misinterpret the directions for recurrence is far too frequent when lesions have been in the chronic stage for months or years. The force of habit lies in the small muscle fasciculi and it requires

1. Much of that which has been said of the after-treatment of rotation lesions, pages 95 and 96, may with some revision be applied to lateral lesions.

constant vigilance to overcome it. While sidebending lesions are almost invariably the result of traumatism, the surrounding tissues are markedly changed in their potentiality. This must not be forgotten; in fact the complete picture of the lesion should always be held before the consciousness when treating these lesions.

Since the cervical area is characterized by both the movements of rotation and sidebending, these types of cervical lesions should under ordinary circumstances be discussed in the same chapter as the thoracic and lumbar lesions of those types; it is for the reason that in the osteopathic treatment of patients cervical lesions are of almost greater importance than any others, that it is necessary to give them the attention of a separate chapter.

A carefully educated sense of touch is the keynote to both osteopathic diagnosis and operative technique. From the very nature of the osteopathic conception, the physical body viewed as a mechanism whose disordered or diseased conditions demand anatomical readjustment, it is imperative that a delicate and educated sense of touch be acquired to order to apply its tenets logically and successfully.—"THE PRACTICE OF OSTEOPATHY," McConnell and Teall.

CHAPTER VI.

CERVICAL LESIONS

The cervical region is the most interesting area of the spine because it is in relation with some of the vital structures of the human body, especially the superior cervical ganglia, the great relay centres for sympathetic fibres to the head. Mechanically speaking, it is the least understood area of the spine. Our great anatomists have failed to comprehend the planes of the articular surfaces of the cervical vertebræ. Ernest Frazer[1] has shown by a drawing that rotation in the cervical area does not take place about a central axis passing through the body of the vertebra but he has not gone beyond that statement. A detailed study of the planes and axes should precede osteopathic consideration.

The body of a typical cervical vertebra, the fourth, is thinner than the body of a thoracic or lumbar vertebra. Its inferior surface is not a flat surface, being concave antero-posteriorly and

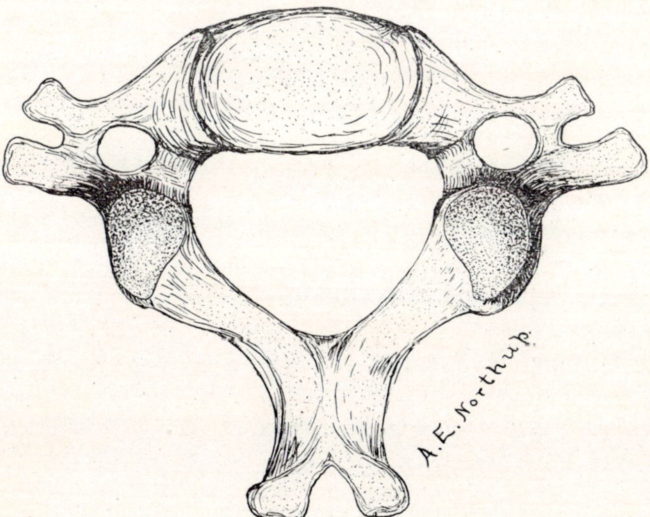

FIG. 41.—Drawing of the sixth cervical vertebra to show the relations of anterior and posterior tubercles and articular facets.

1. Loc. cit.

one-third less deep than transversely wide. Its anterior margin projects as a lip over the superior margin of the fifth vertebral body below. It rests upon an intervertebral disc. It is shallow in comparison with the discs of other regions and is wedge-shaped with the base of the wedge anterior. Due to the shape of the discs the cervical area presents a physiological curve, convex anteriorly. The superior surface of the body of the fifth is transversely concave with lateral margins projecting upward, like lips, a distance of a quarter of an inch. With the lateral margins of the inferior surface of the body of the fourth above, they form diarthrodial joints, the gliding of the inferior surfaces being almost vertically upward and downward upon the inner margins of the lips of the fifth below.[1] It should now be plainly seen that rotation about a central axis is impossible. Due to the elasticity of the nucleus pulposus,[2] there may be slight movement between the bodies in any cervical articulation[3] but not like that of the thoracic joint.

The roots of the arch, the pedicles, of the fourth are short and spring from the lateral aspect of the body. The laminæ are flat and long, meeting at an obtuse angle posteriorly, from which junction projects a bifid spinous process for the attachment of extensor muscles. At the point of union of pedicles and laminæ are developed the articular facets, the upper one projecting upward, backward, and medially, the lower one, downward, forward, and outward. If the articular facets were considered apart from the rest of the vertebra, in the matter of rotation, the axis for the inferior facets would be a line somewhere in the front part of the neck; the axis for the superior facts, a line bisecting the external occipital protuberance. The absurdity of such a proposition appears on the face of it.

The transverse processes are formed of two parts, springing from the body anteriorly and from the arch laterally, united by a bridge of bone which forms thereby the transverse foramen for

1. Morris's "Anatomy", page 226, last paragraph.
2. Morris, loc. cit., page 226, second paragraph.
3. Osteopathically considered, the cervical area is divided into three parts, the atlanto-epistrophic articulation; the articulations of the epistropheus and third, the third-fourth, and the fourth-fifth; the articulations of the fifth-sixth and the sixth-seventh. The seventh cervical is regarded as a thoracic vertebra.

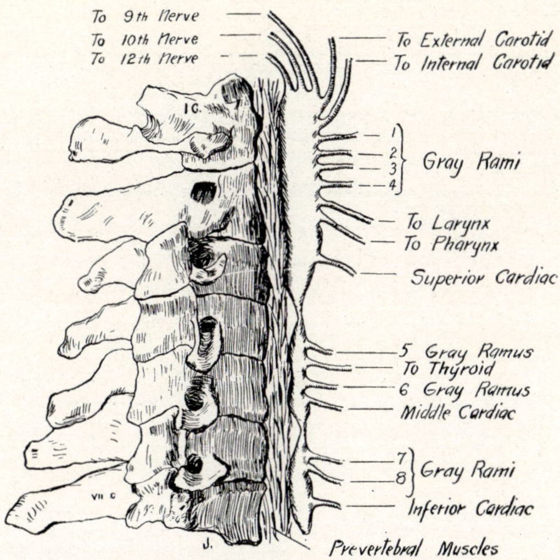

FIG. 42.—Lateral aspect of the cervical area showing the transverse processes and their close relationship to the articular facets just behind them. The three cervical plexuses of the sympathetic system have been sketched anterior to the prevertebral muscles to show the wide-reaching effect of interference by lesion upon this area.

the transmission of the vertebral artery and vein and a sympathetic plexus of nerves. The anterior part, called the costal process because it is the homologue of the rib in the thoracic region,[1] shows a prominence which is termed the anterior tubercle.

The posterior part of the transverse process has been called the posterior tubercle. It projects laterally farther than the anterior tubercle and its posterior surface lies in a horizontal plane less than three-sixteenths of an inch in front of the upper anterior margin of the superior articular facet of the vertebra below. If the inferior facet were to glide backward upon this superior facet, the posterior surface of its posterior tubercle would come in contact[2] almost instantly with the surface of the superior facet above

1. Gray's "Anatomy," page 50, paragraph 2.

2. I am indebted to my student, Mr. George Eddy of the January, 1917, class, for a thorough dissection of the cervical spinal area. Mr. Eddy found that when the coverings of bone and the muscles were deducted from the three-sixteenths of an inch noted above there remained but one-sixteenth of an inch of space through which the inferior facet might glide backward. It is my opinion that osteopathists have not given enough attention to the relation of these bony processes in the consideration of cervical lesions.

mentioned, thus again proving that rotation does not take place upon a central or an oblique axis.

The osteopathist has at his command the means, palpation,[1] of demonstrating that the axis of motion in cervical rotation is a line perpendicular to the surface of the superior articular facet of the lower of the two vertebra in each articulation of the side toward which rotation is made. The axis of motion differs among the different cervical articulations for the reason that as the cervical area merges into the thoracic, the articular surfaces come to resemble those of the adjacent region. The lower cervical area is characterized by sidebending, while the upper cervical area is characterized by rotation.

The lesions of the cervical region are usually rotation or sidebending lesions and from the prominence of the anterior tubercle of the transverse process of the vertebra in lesion, the lesion has been named "anterior on the right" or "anterior on the left." A third cervical anterior on the right may be defined as a lesion in which the third-fourth cervical articulation is immobilized in the position of rotation to the left. A sixth cervical anterior on

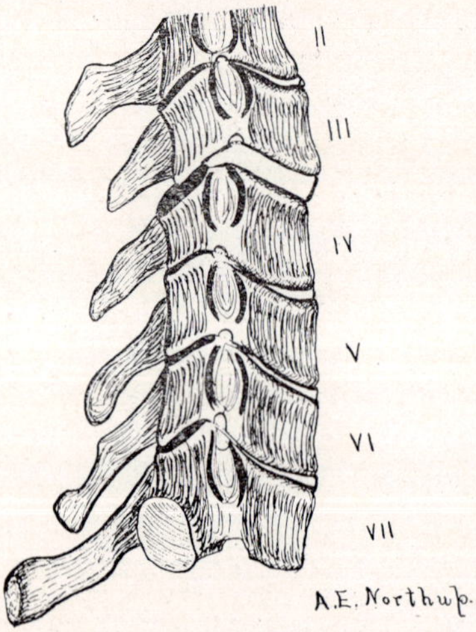

FIG. 43.—Drawing to represent the right lateral view of a right anterior third cervical lesion.

1. Experiment V, page 26.

the right is a lesion in which the sixth-seventh articulation is immobilized in the position of sidebending to the left.[1]

The relation of the anatomical structures in such a lesion would be:

1. Spinous process to the right.[2]
2. The right anterior tubercle of the transverse process of the third in advance of the anterior tubercles of the second and fourth.
3. The left anterior tubercle of the transverse process of the third very slightly posterior in the line of left anterior tubercles which is not usually apparent upon palpation.
4. The vertebral body of the third rotated toward the left slightly with secondary sidetilting upward upon the right and downward upon the left.
5. Intervertebral disc compressed upon the left, stretched and widened upon the right.
6. Axis of motion, a line perpendicular to the left superior articular facet of the fourth cervical vertebra.
7. Intervertebral foramen on the left narrowed, on the right widened vertically.
8. Ligamentous changes.—The right capsular and flava stretched; the right halves of the anterior and posterior longitudinal stretched, the left halves relaxed.
9. Muscles.—The right third-fourth intertransversarii stretched; fasciculi of the scaleni anterior and medius, levator scapulæ, and splenius cervicis attached to the right transverse process of the third cervical vertebra, stretched.

EXPERIMENTAL PALPATION, G.—The patient, B, is assumed to have a right anterior third cervical. According to the manner of palpation in experiment V, page 26, let the radial border of the index finger of each hand rest upon the anterior tubercles of the second, third, and fourth transverse processes, to note any difference that may exist among them.[3] If the third on the right is in lesion, the anterior tubercle of that vertebra will be markedly in advance of the second and fourth tubercles and also in advance when compared with the left anterior tubercle of the third. When the prominence of this tubercle has been determined, the functional

1. Experiment VII, page 28.
2. In the earlier literature of osteopathy, these lesions were called lateral lesions, named according to the side toward which the spinous process seemed turned. Since there has been a more careful study of the differences in bones, the impossibility of diagnosing from a process the direction of whose surface is determined by muscle pull is readily understood. The cervical spinous processes vary in individuals of the same family.
3. The patient should always be asked to hold his head easily erect when cervical palpation is attempted.

test for motion should be made by asking the patient to turn the head to the left, whereupon, if the third were not in lesion but characterized by an anomalous large anterior tubercle, movement would be felt. If however the third is in lesion, there will be no change in the relations of the third and fourth. The second will advance to the line of the third, perhaps, but of the line of anterior tubercles below the second the third will be noticeably anterior. B's head should then be turned to the front, whereupon the anterior tubercles of the two sides will be found equal save for the anterior third. B is asked to turn his head to the right. If movement is felt between the third and fourth tubercles, the third is not in lesion, but if the prominence of the third is in no way lessened by the movement of right rotation, a right anterior lesion is present.

EXPERIMENTAL PALPATION, H.—For the detection of the influence of sidebending upon the lesioned articulation, experiment VII, page 28, should be repeated, and after the plan of experimental palpation, G, above, a determination of the presence of a lesion in a patient supposed to have an anterior fifth cervical on the right may be easily made.

Osteopathists differ in the manner of palpating these lesions. It is possible to detect them, after some experience, by palpating the margins of articular facets posteriorly;[1] by palpating the

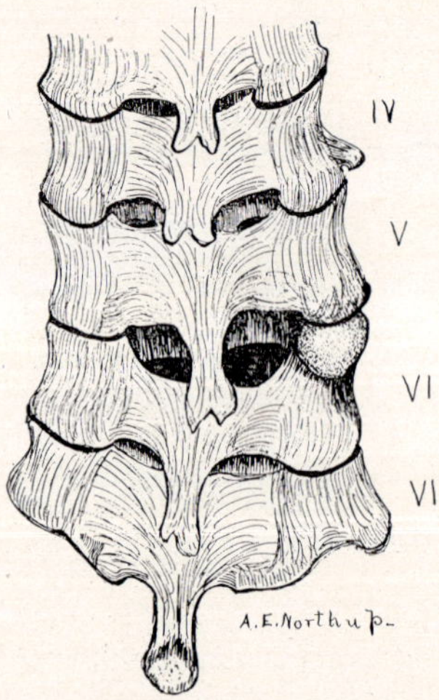

FIG. 44.—Drawing to represent the posterior view, of a right anterior fifth cervical lesion.

1. Method preferred by Dr. H. H. Fryette of Chicago.

lateral surfaces of the transverse processes, or by palpating medially to the anterior tubercles.[1] It requires experience to determine readily which vertebra is in lesion. The axis lacks tubercles upon its transverse processes but these processes after much palpation may be quite readily found. The sixth cervical commonly has exceedingly large tubercles, called from the fact that the carotid artery may be easily compressed against them, the carotid tubercles. By counting upward from these the number of the vertebra in lesion may be determined.

Lesions of the epistropheus may be difficult to diagnose for the reason that often a mass of muscle or connective tissue so surrounds its transverse processes that palpation needs to be skilled to find the surfaces of the transverse processes and to determine whether or not they are in lesion.

Differential diagnosis, when the presence of an anomalous vertebra is suspected, may be made by restriction of motion, the constant sign of lesion. The cervical area is subject to caries and arthritis and the student should exercise care in differentiating these cases[2] by the history of the case, the presence of deformity, and of characteristic symptoms.[3] Cervical lesions are often difficult of diagnosis and obstinate of correction due to the fact that there has been calcareous deposit about the articular processes.

Of the causes producing cervical lesions the commonest are traumatism and infection. The usual traumatisms are forcible twisting or sidebending of the neck. Of the infections causing a secondary inflammation of the cervical articulations, the usual ones are tonsillitis, influenza, diphtheria, scarlet fever, measles, mumps, otitis media, mastoiditis, and acute articular rheumatism. Any distrubance in the blood or nerve supply to the articulation weakens its resistance to active agents. Sudden muscular contractions may cuase a strain of a cervical joint and direct violence may also produce lesion. Acute wryneck is usually followed by

---

1. Method preferred by Dr. H. W. Forbes of Los Angeles.

2. Dr. C. P. McConnell has said recently that diagnostic ability depends upon differentiation of cause from effect. This is particularly true when one wishes to determine the difference in a cervical condition, which might be confused as to whether arthritis or simple chronic rotation lesion with deposit.

3. "Orthopedic Surgery," Royal Whitman, 1910, pg. 46, 129, 131, 133. "Diseases of Infancy and Childhood," L. E. Holt, M. D., 1906 edit., page 903.

one or more cervical subluxations. Faulty posture from ocular defect, sleeping with the head sidebent or twisted, occupations requiring a constant turning of the head, are all predisposing factors in cervical lesion production.

CORRECTIVE MOVEMENTS

THE PRINCIPLES OF CORRECTION FOR CERVICAL LESIONS ARE ROTATION AND SIDEBENDING.

GENERAL RULES.—SINCE ROTATION AND SIDEBENDING ARE CONCOMITANT A CERVICAL LESION MAY BE CORRECTED BY PLACING THE PATIENT IN THE POSITION OF SIDEBENDING AND USING THE MOVEMENT OF ROTATION FOR CORRECTION, OR BY PLACING THE PATIENT IN THE POSITION OF ROTATION AND USING THE MOVEMENT OF SIDEBENDING FOR CORRECTION.[1]

THE ARTICULATING SURFACES MUST RETRACE THE PATH THEY TOOK IN THEIR DISPLACEMENT.[2]

There is no area of the spine where preliminary treatment is so necessary as in the cervical region. The muscles are many, their fasciculi take origin from more than one vertebra usually, and contractions are easily induced by irritation to the supplying nerve. Patients do not relax easily to corrective movements and many suffer from muscular rigidities incident to the chronic condition of the case.[3]

A certain amount of massage may be helpful in relaxation of contracted muscles but the preferred method is a stretching of the tissues by putting the neck through the normal movements of the cervical area, flexion, extension, rotation, and sidebending. The osteopathist should have in mind separation of the origin and insertion of each muscle. In this way a direct longitudinal pull is given to the muscle which tends to overcome its contraction. The separation must be effected slowly, for all hurried, jerky movements defeat their own purpose, relaxation. Nowhere in the application of osteopathic mechanics is quiet action, carefulness in the

1. Whether sidebending or rotation be initiative, the body rotates to the concavity of the curve in the general movement preceding lesion production.
2. This is a general law and applicable in the correction of all joint lesions.
3. Unquestionably relaxation makes the patient ready and secondarily so prepares the tissues that subsequent movements do not serve to lessen his confidence.

application of force, and skill more necessary. The head may be taken in the hands, one on each side, one below the occiput and the other over the forehead, or with one below the occiput and the other grasping the chin, with the object of stretching the cervical region by pulling the head in the direction of the movement desired. The head may be supported by one hand to move it in a desired direction while the other hand about the neck assists. The patient may be seated upon a stool or lying supine upon a table for preliminary treatment.

When the patient has acquired the ability to relax to the general movements of the area, he should then be given the corrective movement by degrees until he relaxes completely so that adjustment shall be absolutely painless and inoffensive. Such preparatory measures may require several visits; they may be accomplished at the first treatment. There is great dissimilarity among patients in this respect.

I. FORBES'[1] MOVEMENT.—Let B be assumed to have a right anterior lesion of the axis. He is asked to sit upon a stool not more than sixteen inches high. O stands behind B and slightly to his left. B is asked to lean back against O who takes hold of B's head with his right hand and lays in on his left forearm, his palm against B's left cheek, the fingers of his hand grasping B's chin, his upper arm resting against the top of B's head. O places his right hand against the right side of B's neck, the metacarpo-phalangeal joint of the index finger against the right lamina of the third cervical vertebra to make of it a fixed point. The web between the index finger and the thumb rests against the right side of B's neck, the fingers of O's hand point directly forward so that they do not touch the neck and induce any reflex contractions by the contact. The palm of O's right hand may be lifted from the side of B's neck or applied to it, as the habit of the practician is.

Maintaining this position, O bends B's head directly over his left shoulder. He then carries his head forward without turning B's face to right or left. Then pushing against the angle of the mandible, he lifts B's chin to the right a distance of about an inch. The purpose of these positions may be explained, thus: sidebending to the left exaggerates the lesion slightly and helps to disengage the surrounding tissues.[2] The head is carried forward in flexion to straighten the cervical curvature that later rotation may be

1. I have chosen to name this movement for Dr. H. W. Forbes for the reason that its efficiency well deserves the appellation.

2. See page 72, line 13.

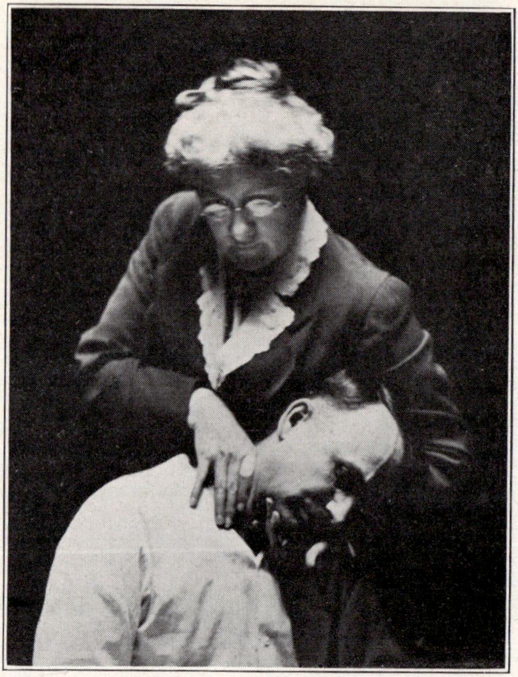

FIG. 45.—Illustrating the first half of the Forbes' movement for the correction of a right anterior axis lesion.

accomplished better as it is when there is less of the physiological curve present; flexion also localizes rotation to the uppermost area of the cervical region.[1] The lifting of the chin is for the purpose of so placing the planes of the articular surfaces of the axis-third articulation that they shall not be jambed by any force directed against them.

Pressure is now placed upon the top of B's head to hold in close apposition the facets of the left side so that movement among them is limited in extent to the purposes of the correction.

B's face is now turned upward and to the right, through an arc measuring about an inch, and then back. This is repeated several times, while the pressure on the top of his head remains unchanged and the fixed point[2] is immovable. When perfect

1. See page 26, paragraph 3.

2. The fixed point is indispensable to the adjustment of the lesion. Without its maintenance, each cervical articulation may be twisted and its articulating surfaces separated by this movement, often resulting in a series of popping sounds.

relaxation is determined by the patient's devitalization of the head, a sudden increase of the turning of the head, to a distance of two or three inches, is made at the same time a slight increase is felt in the pressure exerted by the right hand and the left arm or axilla. This rotation should accomplish a return of the right inferior articular facet of the second cervical to a position of apposition upon the corresponding superior facet of the third, which adjusts the lesion.

Holding the head in the position attained after adjustment has been made, and losing none of the pressure upon the head or at the fixed point, the head is brought over toward the right shoulder in right sidebending. Pressure is repeatedly relaxed and increased upon the top of the head in this position for the purpose of grinding any calcareous deposit that may have formed and also for a stimulative effect upon the elastic fibres of the right capsular ligament and the fasciculi of the muscles that have become atonic.[2]

A slight popping sound[3] usually occurs at the moment preceding adjustment and is probably due to the separation of the parts of the articulating surfaces that had been held immobilized in lesion.

Lesions from the axis to the fourth are corrected as the axis lesion in the above movement, the head in each lower lesion being bent less far to the left side, and the fixed point being changed always to the lamina of the vertebra below the one in lesion. The reverse by position will adjust lesions upon the left side of the cervical region.

II. Approximating Movement.—B is assumed to have a right anterior lesion of the third cervical vertebra. B is asked to lie supine upon the table. O draws him upward until his head extends just beyond the edge of the table and then places a pillow against the top of his head and holds it firmly by pressure with abdomen against the pillow. Rising slightly on his tiptoes, O flexes B's head according to the vertebra that is in lesion. If B has a right anterior axis, O flexes B's head as much as is comfortable. If B has a right anterior sixth cervical, O flexes B's head merely enough to raise it from the table. Flexion localizes rotation in the cervical area; the greater the degree of flexion, the less in extent the number of vertebræ taking part in rotation, from

1. This also stretches the contractured muscles on the opposite side of the neck. Any localized right sidebending or rotation will stretch them.

2. It is usually best to explain in advance to the patient that a popping sound may be heard for many people have erroneous ideas concerning joint sounds. The movement should be absolutely painless to the patient. The amount of force necessary for the adjustment is slight. The frequent fault with beginners is using too much force.

the axis downward. In this movement B is assumed to have a right anterior axis lesion.

O places both hands underneath B's neck, the right hand to make a fixed point of the third cervical vertebra, by pressure against the spinous process and the right lamina or transverse process. O's left hand holds the head under the occiput with the heel of the hand against the parietal or the temporal bone to guide the head in movement.

O sidebends B's head to the right and rotates it slightly to the same side, at the same time maintaining a steady but not painful pressure against the top of his head. The movement is directed toward returning the right inferior facet of the axis backward and downward upon the right superior facet of the third vertebra. Slight relaxation of the pressure is made as the head is returned to the median line but increased again upon repetition of the movement. When relaxation has been secured, by an increase of sidebending and rotation and with no loss of pressure upon the head, adjustment is usually effected.[1]

This movement is exceedingly gentle and to patients who are high-strung or nervous it is well adapted. It may be used in the correction of any of the anterior cervical lesions.

III. UPRIGHT-ROTATION MOVEMENT.—B is assumed to have a right anterior fifth cervical lesion. He sits upon the stool as in movement I, with O standing behind him and slightly to the left. O holds B's head and places his left hand against the lamina of the sixth as in the above movement. B's head is bent slightly to the left. O then rotates B's head directly to the right in an arc of about thirty degrees, at the same time maintaining firmly the fixed point, the sixth vertebra. He repeats the rotation until relaxation is secured and then increases the arc of rotation with a quick movement which should correct the lesion.[2] To hold the adjustment, further movement is necessary. O should maintain the rotation, lift slightly upon B's chin, hold the pressure against the top of his head and sidebend his head to the right at the same time thrusting the sixth cervical vertebra to the left and slightly downward by increasing the pressure against the lamina of that vertebra. This movement of sidebending should be repeated by bringing B's head back to the erect position, not losing the rotation and the pressures and again sidebending it.

This movement is corrective for anterior cervical lesions of the fifth and sixth cervical vertebræ. Movements I and III may

1. A reversing of hands and movements will correct lesions upon the left.
2. Illustrated by figure 46.

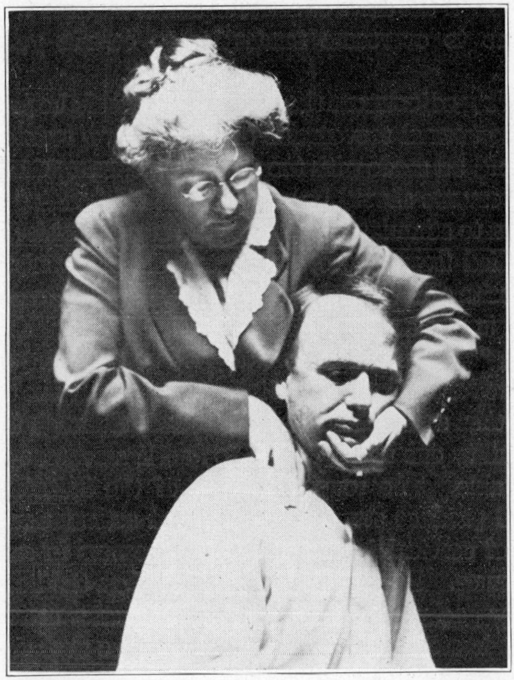

FIG. 46.—Illustrating the position in the upright-rotation movement when the right inferior facet of the fifth is brought to apposition with the corresponding superior facet of the sixth.

be adapted to the supine position by changing the positions of the hand and arm which hold the head, bending slightly over the patient, so that the left forearm may serve to assist in guiding the head in the movements to the right.

AFTER-TREATMENT

The articulations of the cervical area require a very considerable amount of treatment following the adjustment of lesions to maintain the correction. The very flexibility of the cervical region, a necessity in the carriage of the head, makes that area a prey to faulty habits of posture. A constant problem with the human being is holding his head erect. He is unconscious of effort in that direction save when he is asked to change a habit.

He finds himself the slave of attitude and it requires vigilance and perseverence to overcome tendencies to certain positions and movements.

Following adjustment the articulation should be put passively through the normal movements and the active, resistance movements should be made with the physician offering the resistance. These movements should be rotation and sidebending to the side of the lesion to stimulate to activity the muscle fasciculi stretched and atrophied from disuse, to stretch the antagonistic muscles of the opposite side which have become contracted and shortened.

There is a condition in the cervical area which has been termed the "wrecked neck" which may be described as a condition of relaxed articulations. It is unquestionably due to improper treatment that such relaxations are found, although in a case of general debility one might expect to find ligamentous tissues and joints unstable. The rough handling of the imitators of osteopathy will produce strains of the spinal articulations; careless snapping[1] of cervical joints will cause looseness in capsules and limiting tissues. Especially is this true when the limitations of extension or backward movement of the superior articular facets are little understood. The treatment of such a neck should begin with resistance movements in flexion and extension, for nearly all of the flexors and extensors are likewise rotators and lateral flexors. Rarely should adjustment be made until the tissues of the neck are strong enough to hold correction.

Cervical lesions[2] may be corrected in one treatment in a neck that is otherwise strong. Without the proper amount of after-treatment these lesions may recur constantly and both physician and patient think that they are difficult of adjustment. Fifteen treatments should overcome any cervical lesion that is not fixed by deposit.

---

1. The habit of putting a cervical joint upon tension and then "popping" it is one to be condemned in no uncertain language. Students who are mere beginners in osteopathic colleges easily acquire by observation the ability to "crack" a neck and untold detriment often results. Patients who have had adjustments affording instant relief, often twist their necks and jerk them about until joints "give" with the suggestive effect of removal of the irritative cause. Cervical treatment should be mastered by slow processes.

2. A comprehensive article upon the subject appeared in the Journal of the A. O. A., May, 1909, page 385, from the pen of Dr. H. W. Forbes.

COUNTERBALANCING LESIONS

When a cervical lesion is present, there may be detected a lengthening of the side of the neck upon which the lesion is found, by reason of the immobilization of the inferior facet in a position forward and upward upon the superior facet below. In consequence of this lesion, the crown of the head will be tilted and turned slightly toward the side opposite the lesion. To overcome this attitude it will be necessary to increase the height of the other side of the neck by a secondary cervical lesion below or by a turning or lateral bending of the head toward the side of the primary lesion.

A cervical lesion may itself be secondary to an occipital lesion above and in such a case the indicated treatment is first adjustment of the primary lesion, followed by correction of the secondary lesion, should it persist, and close attention to resistance exercises. Cervical curvatures,[1] in a large percentage of cases, are compensatory in character, the primary cause being an occipital or atloid lesion. Habit[2] is a predisposing factor of great importance in these patients.

1. See page 47, line 5.

2. The interesting case of Mr. C. E. Moyer of the June, 1916, Class, may be cited in this connection. Mr. Moyer has been a professional baseball pitcher. At the close of each season, his cervical area has presented lesions which could be explained by reason of his position on the diamond He has had a slight cervical curvature, convex to the right, made necessary by almost constantly watching the first base; in addition he has had a rotation of the occiput and atlas to the right, the result of turning to throw the ball. The struggle for supremacy among the muscles of the neck has brought among them an unusual division in action.

Bibliography: Cunningham, ibid., pg. 90-93, 305-309, 368, 392, 438-446, 467-470.

Deaver, ibid., I, pg. 372, 377, 400-407, 412-424.

Frazer, ibid., pg. 15-24.

Gray, ibid., pg. 49-53, 268-273.

Morris, ibid., pg. 31-35, 224-232, 320, 321, 353, 356, 414-419, 502.

Scudder's "Treatment of Fractures," 1914, pg. 644-651.

CHAPTER VII

SACRO-ILIAC LESIONS

One of the earliest discoveries of the founder of the science of osteopathy was that the sacro-iliac joint is a freely movable articulation and therefore subject to subluxation. This joint had been termed by anatomists immovable but later, when Sir Richard Quain, the great English surgeon, called attention to the manner in which the sacrum was suspended between the ossa coxæ, the sacro-iliac articulation was decided to be slightly movable and was classified among the amphiarthrodia. About twenty years after Dr. A. T. Still had been adjusting subluxations of the innominates and fully ten years after he had taught the osteopathic methods of reduction for these subluxations, followers of the regular school of medicine began research into the action of this joint, with the noticeable result that there is scarcely a medical text in gynecology, obstetrics, or orthopedic surgery today but which speaks of strain of these articulations; the methods therein offered for their correction are chiefly through rest, mechanical supports, and the use of weights.

Not only can the researches of the osteopathic scientists now offer a more thorough knowledge of the sacro-iliac articulation but they can give reasons for differences in pelvic inclination, offer etiologic causes for pelvic congestion, and explain the foundation for the faulty attitudes of the straight spine, flat chest, and round shoulders.

Bibliography: Marion E. Clark, ibid., pg. 301-330.
Cunningham, ibid., pg. 96-99, 228-238, 334-339, 301.
Dunlop, "Amer. Jour. Ortho. Surg.", July 1907, pg. 151.
H. W. Forbes, "Jour. of A. O. A.", Aug. 1909, Apr. and May, 1910.
Ernest Frazer, ibid., pg. 37-43, 115-134.
Goldthwait and Osgood, "Bos. Med. and Sur. Jour.", May 25 and June 1, 1905.
Gray, ibid., pg. 58-62, 207-220, 289-295.
Lovett, ibid., pg. 5-6.
C. P. McConnell, in "Jour. of A. O. A.", Nov. and Dec., 1912.
McConnell and Teall, ibid., pg. 57-60, 87-90.
Morris, ibid., pg. 39-42, 169-177, 232-240.
Tasker, "Principles of Osteopathy", 1913 edit., pg. 269-282, 461-470.
Royal Whitman, ibid., pg. 146-148.

The pelvis is formed by the union of four bones, the sacrum, the two innominates or hip-bones, and the coccyx. It has four joints in adult life, the two sacro-iliac articulations, the symphysis pubis, and the sacrococcygeal. It is divided into two parts at the junction of the planes,[1] the promontory of the sacrum, and the upper margin of the pubes. The larger and upper cavity is called the false pelvis, the lower and smaller, the true pelvis. The upper opening of the true pelvis is termed the inlet, the lower opening the outlet. The pelvis is spoken of as a bony girdle or basin which to the unthinking mind might convey the idea of solidity with joints subject to little change. On the contrary, the two greater joints of the pelvis, the sacro-iliac, are now classed among the diarthrodia, freely moving articulations.

The sacrum is wedge-shaped from above downward, its base articulating with the fifth lumbar vertebra; it is also wedge-shaped from before backward, a fact that makes clear the statement that the sacrum is held suspended between the innominates by strong ligaments instead of completing the bony girdle as the keystone caps the arch.

The ligaments of the sacro-iliac joint are the anterior sacro-iliac, the posterior sacro-iliac, and the interosseous sacro-iliac, the last-named the most important ligament of the articulation. It consists of very strong fibres of uneven length passing from the rough area on the ilium posterior and adjacent to the auricular surface, medially and downward, to be attached to the posterior surface of the upper two segments of the sacrum. The ligaments of the articulation are in effect capsular ligaments with specially developed bands of strength, holding the surfaces opposed so that dislocation may be prevented yet free movement permitted.

The sacrum and ischium are connected by two ligaments of great strength which limit the motion of the joint, the sacro-tuberous and sacro-spinous,[2] both of which are attached to the posterior aspect and lateral margins of the sacrum and coccyx, and the first has also an attachment to the posterior inferior spine of the ilium. The sacro-tuberous ligament is inserted into the medial

1. The iliopectineal lines.
2. Old terminology, greater and lesser sacro-sciatic ligaments.

border of the tuberosity of the ischium; the sacro-spinous into the inner surface and borders of the spine of the same bone.

The pubic articulation is an amphiarthrosis, has slight mobility, and is influenced by lesions of the sacro-iliac joints.

EXPERIMENTAL PALPATION, I.—Ask the subject to lie upon the table upon his face, with his hands resting palm downward upon the table beside his shoulders. Ask him to raise his torso gradually backward from the table until only the lower part of the abdomen rests upon the table. He must be instructed to raise his body by the power on the muscles of his arms, so that the extensor muscles of the back shall remain relaxed. O places his thumbs upon the coccygeal end of the sacrum, his index fingers upon the base of the sacrum close to the over-lapping surface of the ilium, the middle fingers upon the posterior superior spines of the innominates. While B rests upon the table, O palpates very carefully the relations of the surfaces his thumb and fingers rest upon, as to planes, distances apart, etc. When B reaches the amount of extension asked, O should note that the coccygeal end of the sacrum is below the horizontal level of the first position; that the index fingers are more nearly at a level with the middle fingers, and that there is a slight increase of distance between the middle fingers. B is asked to return to the prone position. Just before his body rests against the table O should be able to note the motion that takes place in the sacro-iliac articulations. There must be no mistaking of the contraction of the erector spinæ muscles for actual movement in these articulations and for this reason B must be trained to keep his extensor muscles relaxed while he raises his body by the muscular strength of his arms.

EXPERIMENTAL PALPATION, J.—Ask the subject, B, to sit upon the end of the table, O sitting upon a stool behind him. An assistant,[1] C, may stand in front of B, his hands under B's axillæ to support him. O places his thumbs and fingers as in the above experiment. O bends his head forward to support the weight of B's trunk when B moves backward in extension, unless C is able to hold B's weight. B is asked to bend forward in much flexion. O should now observe that the coccygeal end of the sacrum has become prominent posteriorly, that the levels of the index and middle fingers differ markedly, that the middle fingers are less far apart than in the prone position in the last experiment. B is asked to carry his torso back in extension, or C is instructed to support B as B leans backward. B's upper thoracic area comes

1. An assistant is required when a flexible subject is not easily obtained. Any person who understands how to relax and who is not obese will be a suitable subject for experimental palpation.

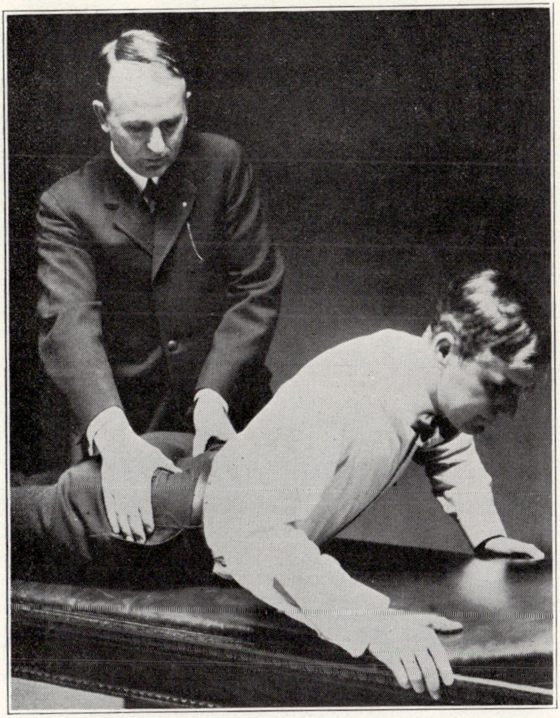

Fig. 47.—Illustrating a manner of palpating for motion in the sacro-iliac articulations. The palmar surfaces of the thumbs rest across the adjacent surfaces of the posterior superior iliac spines and the posterior surface of the sacrum.

to the level of O's head and he rests against O's head. O should observe that the relative condition of the palpated surfaces change with the movement. The coccygeal end of the sacrum moves forward, the middle fingers separate, the index fingers approach the level of the middle fingers, thus proving that the axis of motion for the sacro-iliac joints is a line which passes through each articular surface at its central point and through the second sacral segment.

Experimental Palpation, K.—Ask the subject, B, to stand upon the floor with his feet several inches apart. O sits behind him upon a high stool and places his thumbs against the margins of the ilia, the tips of his thumbs resting upon the posterior, adjacent surface of B's sacrum. B is then asked to bend forward from the waist. O should observe that the tips of his thumbs move slightly forward in relation to the first joint of his thumbs

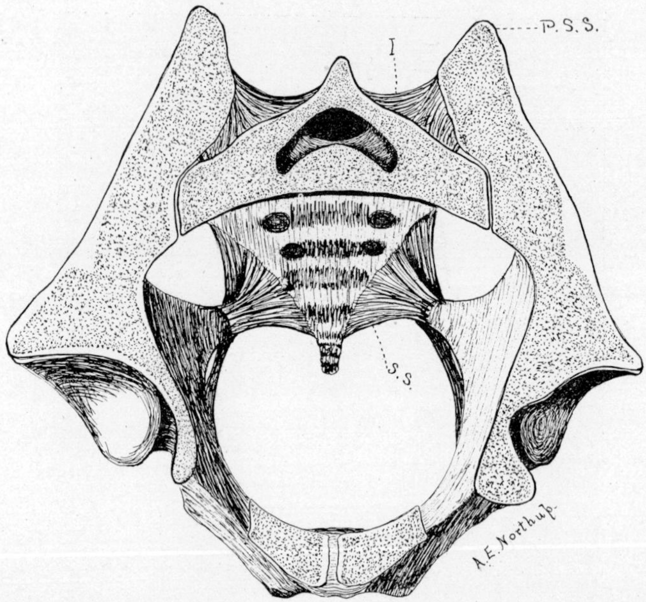

FIG. 48.—Cross section through the second sacral segment of the pelvis, as seen from above, showing the inlet, outlet, articulations, and ligaments. P. S. S., the posterior superior spine of the ilium. I, The interosseous and posterior sacro-iliac ligament. S. S., sacro-sciatic ligaments, great and lesser.

which rest against the ilia and also that the distance between the ilia is lessened. B is asked to resume the erect position and bend backward from the waist in extension. It may now be noted that the tips of the thumbs move backward until they are nearly in the same vertical plane as the first joints.

These movements should be repeated until O has demonstrated for himself the character and amount of the motion in B's sacro-iliac articulations.

A consideration of each movement in detail is important. When the base of the sacrum moves forward in flexion, the movement is limited by the sacro-sciatic ligaments which being attached below to the end of the sacrum and the coccyx, are stretched taut when those bones move upward and backward. If palpation is made through the rectum, the tautness of these ligaments is easily demonstrated. They may be called the check-ropes of the sacro-iliac articulations.

If with a steel tape[1] measurement has been made of the distance between the two posterior superior spines of the ilia, a second measurement made after flexion will show exactly that the posterior superior spines are closer together than in the upright position of the normal pelvis. If a fixed point on the posterior surface of the sacrum be chosen, as for example the second sacral spinous process, and measurements made from it to each posterior superior iliac spine in each of these positions, the same observation may be made, namely, that the superior spines move toward each other slightly in flexion of the sacrum.

With a pelvic model having movable articulations, when flexion of the sacrum is produced, there are noticeable changes in the pelvic outlet and inlet: the tuberosities of the ischii move outward; the outlet is widened laterally and antero-posteriorly; the anterior superior spines of the ilia are less widely separated, thus reducing the broad diameter of the false pelvis; the lumbo-

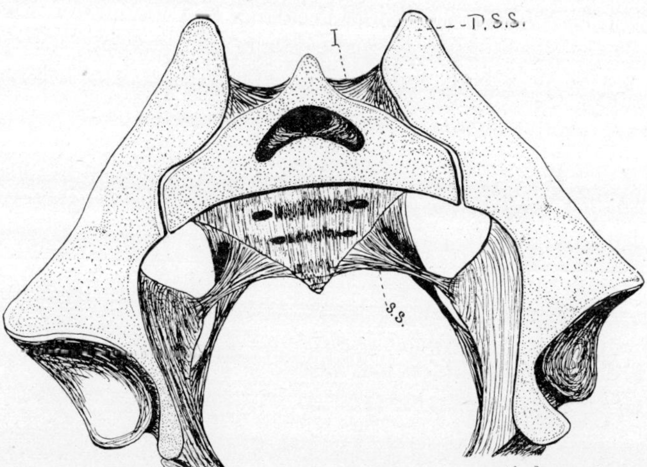

FIG. 49.—Cross section through the second sacral segment showing the change in the diameters of the outlet of the pelvis when a flexion lesion of the sacrum is present.

1. A narrow steel tape is best for there is little chance of its being injured by use. A cotton or linen tape may be stretched so that its measurement is quite inaccurate. A tape having the metric system upon one side and the English upon the other is to be preferred.

sacral angle projects forward into the false pelvis, and the antero-posterior diameter of the inlet is narrowed.

Passing in review all these facts, it is possible to grasp what the motion between the articular surfaces of the sacrum and ilia is. Rotation is proved by the upward movement of the inferior extremity of the sacrum and by the forward movement of the base of the sacrum occurring at one and the same time. Gliding, which is concomitant with rotation, is proved by the separation of the ischial tuberosities and by the narrowing of the distance between the anterior superior spines. Upon the strength of the posterior sacro-iliac ligaments depends the prevention of anterior dislocation in this position, which the weight transmitted from the body above through the base of the sacrum tends to produce.

FLEXION LESION OF THE SACRUM

Immobilization, partial or complete, may take place in the pelvis in flexion of the sacrum.[1] Such a lesion is spoken of as a flexion lesion of the sacrum or as bilaterally posterior innominate lesions. Its usual cause is debility, weakness of the flexor muscles, undue contraction of the extensors from irritation, faulty habits of posture, improper clothing, and rachitis. It is most frequently found in children and is accompanied by round shoulders and sunken chest.[2] The lumbar area may or may not go forward in lordosis[3] and the abdomen usually protrudes.

When a flexion lesion of the sacrum is thought to be present from the appearance of the patient as above described, the diagnosis may be established by the following signs:

1. Limited motion in the sacro-iliac articulations.
2. Decreased distance between the posterior superior spines when compared with the average which is three and one-half inches.
3. Taut sacro-sciatic ligaments.
4. The presence of counterbalancing lesions, most commonly a lumbar lordosis.

1. This lesion has been termed the anterior sacrum.
2. Cf. Lovett, ibid., Chap. XIII, page 178-180, 182.
3. Lordosis is the term for an increase in the lumbar curve, convex anteriorly.

CORRECTIVE MOVEMENTS

THE PRINCIPLES OF CORRECTION FOR A FLEXION LESION OF THE SACRUM ARE EXTENSION OF THE SACRUM OR FLEXION OF BOTH INNOMINATES.

Since these lesions are of gradual production, correction must proceed slowly with attention to the removal of the cause when that lies in removable conditions, as in faulty posture or unhygienic surroundings.

Preliminary treatment is of much advantage in these cases for the muscles of the lumbar area of the spine and the thigh are often unduly contracted and require relaxation. Any unbalance of the pelvis will cause marked deviations from the normal in the spine above or in the muscles which hold the pelvis upright. The effects of unbalance, wherever found, must be overcome as early in the treatment of the case as possible.

I. EXTENSION-HOLDING MOVEMENT.—Let B, who is assumed to have a flexion lesion of the sacrum, lie prone upon the table. O standing beside the table places his hands upon the posterior superior spinous processes of the ilia and presses firmly against these while B by lifting himself with his arms carries his trunk backward in extension. When B has reached the amount of extension desirable, O should place his hands, one over the other, against the lower part of the sacrum, below the segment through which passes the axis of rotation, and exert firm pressure while B returns to the prone position. The movements B executes should be performed slowly.

Any of the corrective movements for a posterior innominate lesion may be used in the correction of the flexion sacral lesion by giving the movement as though for lesions of both innominates.[1]

Material assistance may be had from the patient in the overcoming of this lesion by the practice of extension at home and also by taking the creeping exercises, before recommended.[2] As soon as the sacro-iliac articulations have normal motion and the posture has markedly improved, the patient should be entered in a reputable gymnasium for a thorough course especially directed to

---

1. See page 146.
2. See page 41, footnote 1. The patient should creep directly ahead instead of in a circle.

the development of the muscular system and respiratory improvement.

SACRAL EXTENSION

When the base of the sacrum moves backward in extension, the movement is limited by the interposition of the anterior surface of that bone, the base of the second wedge of the sacrum. Dislocation is therefore an impossibility in this direction. If the distance between the posterior superior spines of the ilia is measured and compared with the same distance in the normal upright position, it will be found to be greater in extension, therefore it is proved that the ilia glide outward and forward when the sacrum rotates backward; simultaneously the ischii will glide backward and inward. As the result of these changes, the false pelvis is broadened laterally, the distance between the anterior superior spines is greater, the inlet of the true pelvis will be widened in both diameters, the outlet of the pelvis will be narrowed correspondingly, and the sacro-sciatic ligaments will be relaxed.

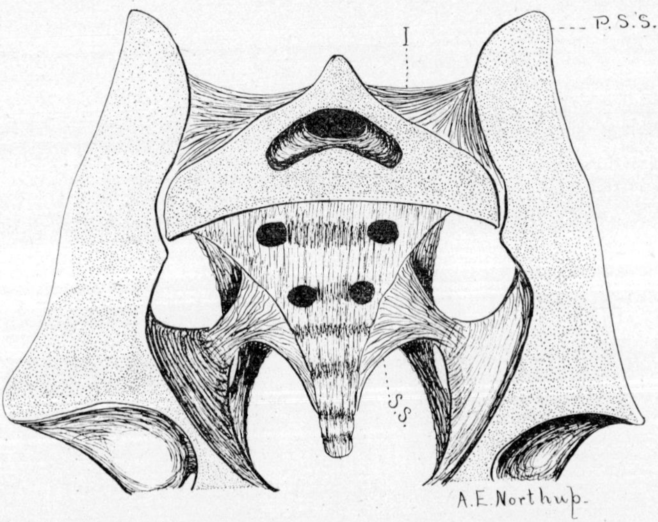

FIG. 50.—Cross section through the second sacral segment of the sacrum, when an extension lesion of the sacrum is present. P. S. S., posterior superior spine. I, interosseous and posterior sacro-iliac ligament. S. S. sacro-sciatic ligaments. The changed diameter of the pelvic outlet is shown.

EXTENSION LESION OF THE SACRUM

Immobilization of the sacro-iliac joints may take place with the sacrum in the position of extension. Its causation is debility, infectious diseases, especially pneumonia, injuries to the spine, the slouched position in sitting, especially when sitting is accompanied with continuous jarring as in riding in conveyances day after day,[1] weakness of the extensor muscles, contraction of the flexors, a shifting of the line of gravity backward from its wonted plane in front of the sacro-iliac joints and the greater part of the vertebral bodies. Tuberculosis in adults with the secondary changes that take place in posture may predispose to strain of the sacro-iliac articulations.

The appearance of a patient who has this lesion is characteristic, for there is present a compensatory straightening of the spine above with a secondary flattening of the thorax. Frequent allusion has been made in medical literature to this attitude and it has been termed the "flat back".[2] In osteopathic literature it is spoken of as "the straight spine and the flat chest". The scapulæ are often winged, the antero-posterior diameter of the thorax is lessened, the transverse, widened.[3]

The significance of the extension lesion of the sacrum can be comprehended only when with a pelvic model in hand, one may demonstrate the narrowing of the outlet that is thus produced and realize what a bearing it would have upon the health of the pelvic tissues and also what a hindrance it would offer to parturition. When the sacro-sciatic ligaments become lax, the soundness of the pelvic floor is endangered, it sags, and congestion results, followed naturally by inflammation of some of the pelvic viscera, the prostate gland, uterus and appendages, rectum, or bladder.

An almost constant symptom of sacral lesion is backache. Nervous disturbances follow rigidity of any articulation which directly or indirectly supports the spinal cord, hence, immobiliza-

1. I am indebted to Dr. Lew A. May for calling my attention to the effects of fatigue and riding upon the ligamentous and muscular tone of the articulation with the subsequent extension lesion of the sacrum. Dr. May has also offered one of the corrective movements which follow.

2. See Lovett, ibid., pg. 181.

3. A fuller discussion of the thoracic changes will be found in the following chapter.

tion of the sacrum, partial or complete, or of one sacro-iliac joint, predisposes to nervous maladies for with each step an irritative jar shocks the delicate nervous tissues above.

The diagnosis of an extension lesion is established by the following signs:

1. Restricted movement in both sacro-iliac articulations.
2. Flattening of the innominates posteriorly.
3. Widening of the distance between the posterior superior spines in comparison with the average measurement between these processes.
4. Relaxed sacro-sciatic ligaments.
5. The presence of counterbalancing lesions; the straight spine, which is characterized by a posterior lumbar area, a flat dorsal area, and depressed ribs.

CORRECTIVE MOVEMENTS

The principles of correction for an extension lesion of the sacrum are flexion of the sacrum or extension of both innominates.

Preliminary treatment may be given before correction of the lesion is attempted. Each innominate should be moved in an attempt to stretch the ligaments of the sacro-iliac articulation. The muscles of the hip-joint should be stretched passively and the lumbar area should receive some attention. Since the lumbar vertebræ have moved backward, they should be given extension.

II. Hamstring Movement.—The patient, B, is assumed to have an extension lesion of the sacrum. He is asked to sit with his feet outstretched upon the table. The pull of the hamstring muscles will fix both innominates. O stands beside him, places one hand across B's thighs just above the knees, the other against B's spine in the lower dorsal area. He holds B's legs to the table at the same time bending him forward toward his knees. The tension upon the sciatic nerve prevents any marked flexion but the movement may afford sufficient motion between the innominates and the sacrum to effect a correction of the lesion after many repetitions.

The patient should practice this movement at home between treatments.

III. Acetabular Leverage Movement.—B is assumed to have a sacral extension lesion. He is asked to lie supine upon the table, and flex his knees resting his feet upon the table. O instructs an assistant, C, to separate B's knees to an angle of about sixty degrees and then to carry the thighs so that they will make with the horizontal plane of the supine body an obtuse angle of about one hundred twenty degrees, or an acute angle with the plane of the table beneath of sixty degrees.[1] He is instructed to place his hands in front of the knees to direct pressure along the shaft of the femur toward the acetabulum.

O stands at the right of B and faces B's feet. O reaches across the table with his left hand and passes it under B's left hip with the purpose of grasping the tuberosity of the left ischium, resting his forearm at the same time strongly against the left iliac crest. With his right hand he takes hold of B's right tuberosity and presses against the right ilium with the forearm. At the time that C directs strong pressure against B's knees, O attempts to pull apart the tuberosities and push medially and backward against the ilia.

It is often helpful to place a small hard pillow under the lumbar area as low as the base of the sacrum, to assist in forcing the base into flexion.

This movement brings out the fact that in an articulation it is often possible to use either bone of that joint as the power arm of a lever.

IV. ISCHIAL SEPARATING MOVEMENT.—Ask the patient, B, to lie prone across the table so that his legs drop off on one side and his head and shoulder girdle on the other side. An assistant, C, puts pressure against the base of the sacrum above the second sacral segment. O puts the heel of each hand against the medial surface of the tuberosity of each ischium to push the tuberosities outward and downward while C holds firmly the base of the sacrum as if to flex that bone forward. This movement should be repeated five or six times at each treatment.

Since the lesion is of gradual production, with counterbalancing changes in posture developing at the same time, there is no open sesame to an immediate correction. The fibres of the lowest fasciculi of the sacro-spinalis (erector spinæ, O. T.) are stretched and atrophied; the complexity of action of the upper divisions of the same muscle is disturbed, and thereby one of the greatest factors in the maintenance of good position becomes inoperative. Tone must be restored to enable it to perform its part in holding

1. In explanation of femur leverage affecting movement in the sacro-iliac articulation it may be pointed out that the acetabulum is diagonally anterior and inferior to the axis of motion.

the body upright and in regaining the normal position of the line of gravity. These patients require considerable tonic treatment and their cooperation must be secured in keeping a careful guard upon themselves that they shall not return into faulty habits of attitude. They need to be taught how to stand, how to sit, how to breathe, and how to curb their ambitions until the physical body is equal to the tasks they have appointed unto themselves. Following the overcoming of the extension lesion of the sacrum, the straight spine, and the flat chest, the patients should pursue for a long time gymnastic work of the general kind to keep a balance of power in the muscular system.

EXTENSION OF THE OS COXÆ

Since the sacrum is the movable bone in the sacro-iliac articulation, extension of the innominate is accomplished by prevention of its participation in the general movement of flexion upon the heads of the femurs. When the sacrum and the other innominate move, the one held immobilized becomes strained at the articulation and a lesion, called the posterior innominate, results.

EXPERIMENTAL PALPATION, L.—Choose a subject, B, who has flexible sacro-iliac articulations, and ask him to sit upon the table with his right ischium upon the table, the right leg outstretched and slightly lateral to the right of a line perpendicular to the mesial plane of the body; let his left ischium and leg be free of the table, the weight resting easily upon the toes of the left foot which should rest upon the floor or a stool. An assistant, C, standing to the right of B, may place his right hand on B's thigh above the knee, pressing it down upon the table while with his left hand against the lower thoracic vertebræ of B's spine, he carries B forward in flexion and holds him there while O makes careful palpation of the posterior surfaces of the ilia and the sacrum. O should find that the posterior superior spinous process of the right innominate seems more prominent than the left one. He should also notice by comparison that the distance between that spinous process and a definite point upon the sacrum is less than the distance between that same point and the posterior superior spinous process of the left innominate. With a steel tape in hand he should confirm his determinations by palpation.

Let B resume the erect position, either standing or sitting, and measurements taken in the same way will show that in the experiment the right ilium glided backward and medially upon the sacrum at the sacro-iliac articulation.

This experiment proves that when the right innominate is fixed as by the pull of the hamstring muscles, flexion of the sacrum and the other innominate, as one bone, upon the immobilized innominate, produces experimentally the posterior innominate lesion.[1] Strain or any other causative factor may in this manner produce the lesion.

A posterior innominate lesion is a subluxation of the sacro-

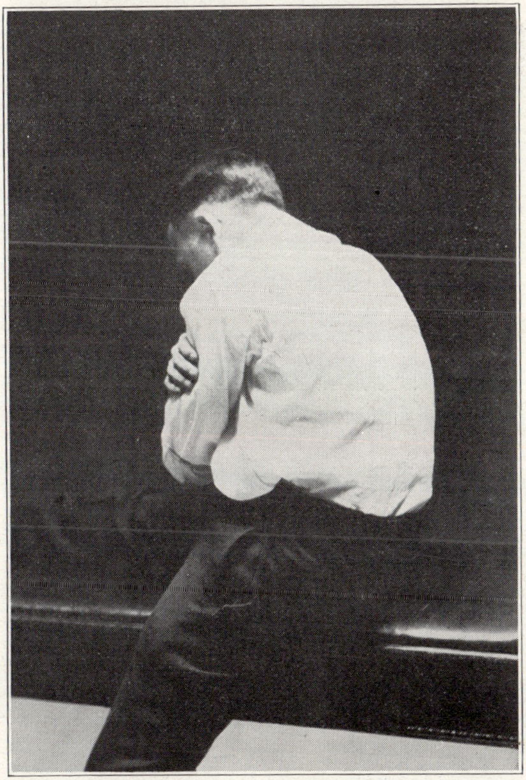

Fig. 51.—Illustrating the experimental production of a posterior innominate lesion.

1. This lesion should most properly be termed an extension lesion of the innominate but the time does not seem to be right for this innovation.

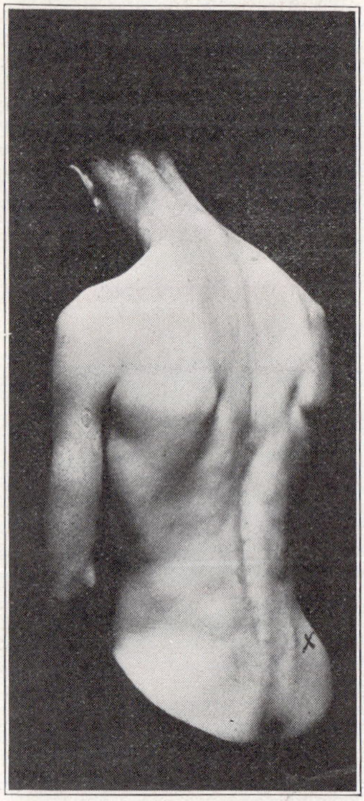

FIG. 52.—Patient with marked evidence of a posterior innominate lesion on the right side.

iliac joint in which the articulation is immobilized in a position of flexion of the sacrum upon one innominate or of the innominate in extension upon the sacrum.

EXAMINATION OF A PATIENT

It is to be assumed that the patient, B, presents himself with symptoms[1] which would lead to the supposition that he has a right posterior innominate lesion, and that upon applying the test[2] for motion, none is found in the right sacro-iliac articulation.

1. Pelvic disturbances, sciatica, orchitis, weak ankle, flat foot, metatarsalgia, varicose veins.
2. See page 129.

B is asked to bare the lower part of his back for inspection. If the lesion is present, it is usual for the right posterior superior spinous process of the innominate to be markedly prominent in the plane of the back. Palpation for comparison of the two posterior superior spinous processes of the ilia shows that the one in lesion is more prominent posteriorly than the other; that in the matter of level, horizontally considered, it is lower than the left.

B is asked to stand and palpation is made of the upper borders of the pubes; when lesion is present, the right pubic bone is slightly higher and a little backward of the other. Palpation per rectum will show that the right sacro-tuberous and sacro-spinous ligaments are taut.

With a steel tape, measurements should be made as in the experiment[1] above to show that the right superior spinous process

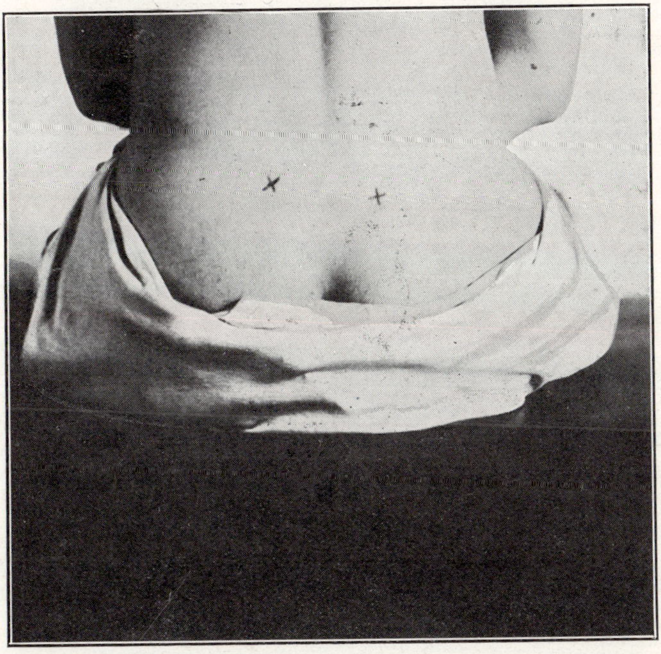

FIG. 53.—Patient with a right posterior innominate, showing the relative heights of the posterior superior spines by the crosses.

1. Experimental palpation, L, page 138.

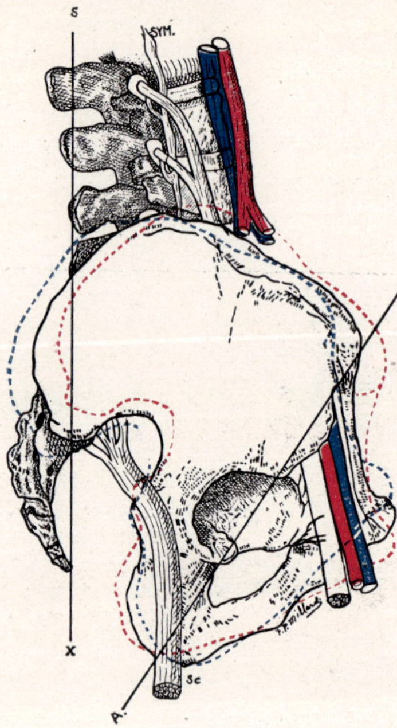

FIG. 54.—Side view of the innominate in its normal position in relation to the sacrum. The dotted lines indicate the directions in which this bone is most likely to be misplaced. The blue dotted line indicates the position the os coxæ would take in a posterior lesion; the red, in an anterior lesion.—(F. P. MILLARD.)

is nearer to a definite point upon the posterior surface of the sacrum in the mid-line than is the left.

In the absence of other lesions, such as curvature, ankylosis of the hip, muscular contracture, etc., there are certain auxilliary signs that are ordinarily present in a case having a posterior innominate lesion. They are not reliable when considered alone and no lesion should be diagnosed without the other signs being present. Both legs should be flexed, extended, rotated, and circumducted before the first of these signs should be sought. The legs may then be brought together upon the table and the length of the heels compared. The one on the side of the posterior innominate will usually be shorter.

If the distance between a definite point upon the sternum and each anterior superior spinous process be measured, it will be found that the distance to the innominate in lesion is less. The distance to the internal malleolus of the same side will be less than the distance to that of the other ankle.

Tenderness and pain upon pressure is a fairly constant symptom but as pain is often due to sensations referred from viscera of lower sensibility,[1] it has not diagnostic accuracy.[2]

Upon the presence of the following unvarying signs may diagnosis be made:

1. Restricted motion in the joint.
2. Prominence of the posterior superior spinous process.
3. Distance from that process to the second sacral spinous process is less than the distance between the same two points upon the left.
4. Right sacro-sciatic ligaments taut.

CORRECTIVE MOVEMENTS

THE PRINCIPLES OF CORRECTION FOR A POSTERIOR INNOMINATE LESION ARE EXTENSION OF THE SACRUM OR FLEXION OF THE INNOMINATE.

GENERAL RULES.—ALL MOVEMENTS MUST CARRY THE BONE THAT IS USED AS A LEVER IN ROTATION ABOUT THE AXIS OF MOTION,

---

1. Henry Head, "On Disturbances of Sensation" in "Brain", 1893, vol. xvi, p. 1; also in sequent numbers, 1894, 1896, 1900, etc.
2. Richard C. Cabot, "Differential Diagnosis," 1912, W. B. Saunders Co., publishers, presents a masterly review of pain as a diagnostic sign.

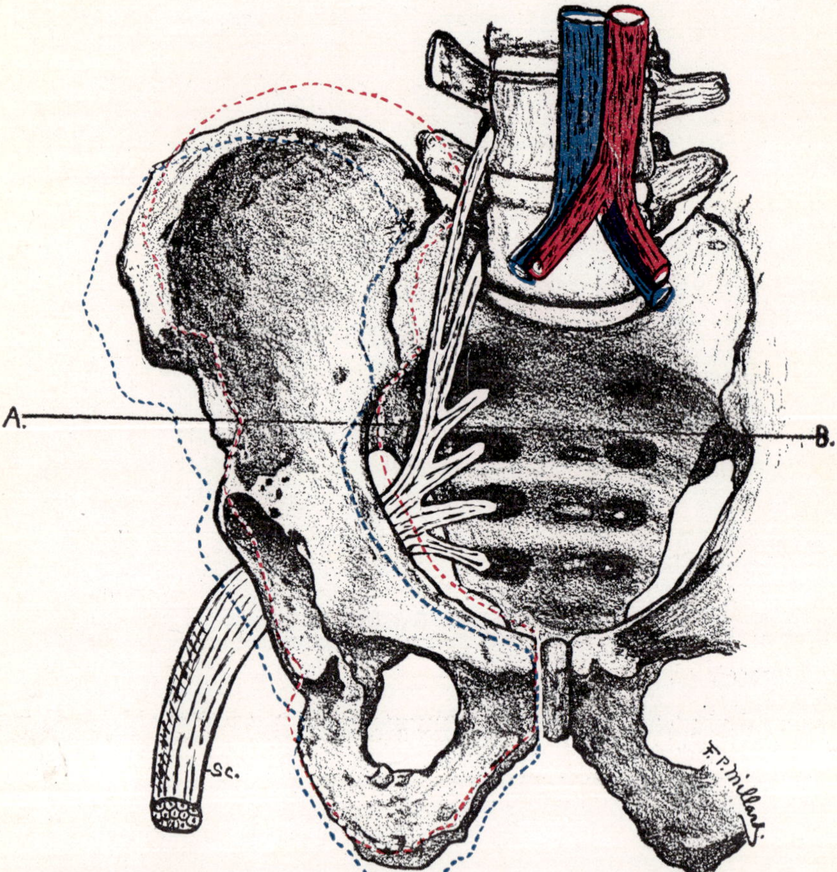

FIG 55.—Anterior view of the pelvis with the innominate in normal position. A.B. is the transverse axis upon which the innominate glides. The red dotted line indicates the position which the innominate would assume in a posterior lesion; the blue dotted line, an anterior innominate lesion.—(F. P. MILLARD.)

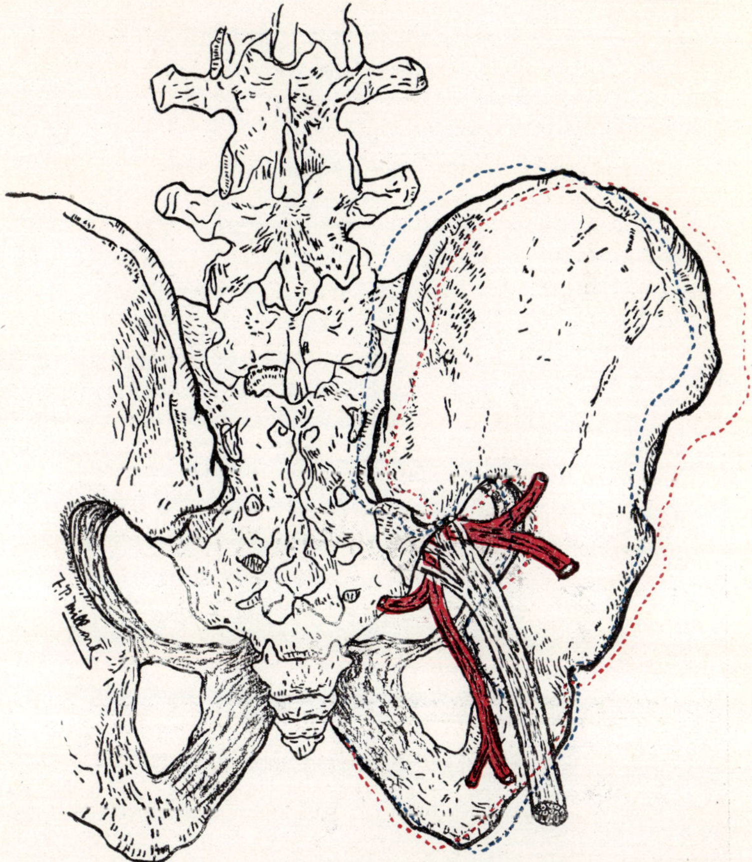

FIG. 56—Posterior view of the ossa coxæ in their normal relationship to the sacrum. The dotted lines show the innominate rotated forward and backward on the transverse axis which passes through the second sacral segment. (F. P. MILLARD.)

A TRANSVERSE ONE INTERSECTING THE SACRO-ILIAC ARTICULAR SURFACES AND THE SECOND SACRAL SEGMENT.

THE DIRECTION OF THE PLANES OF THE ARTICULATING SURFACES MUST BE KEPT BEFORE THE MIND CONTINUALLY THAT NO MOVEMENT SHALL JAM THESE PLANES.

Flexion of the innominate is a movement of rotation and secondary outward gliding, and the mechanical principle involved is that of the wheel and axle. The points of attack about the innominate are the most advantageous leverages by which this movement may be made effective in adjusting lesions of the sacro-iliac joint.

For the correction of the posterior innominate lesion, the following points of attack may be noted: the tuberosity of the ischium, the posterior superior spinous process and the adjacent crest of the ilium, the anterior border of the ilium through the following muscles, sartorious, direct head of the rectus femoris, tensor fasciæ latæ, and the acetabulum by its contact with the

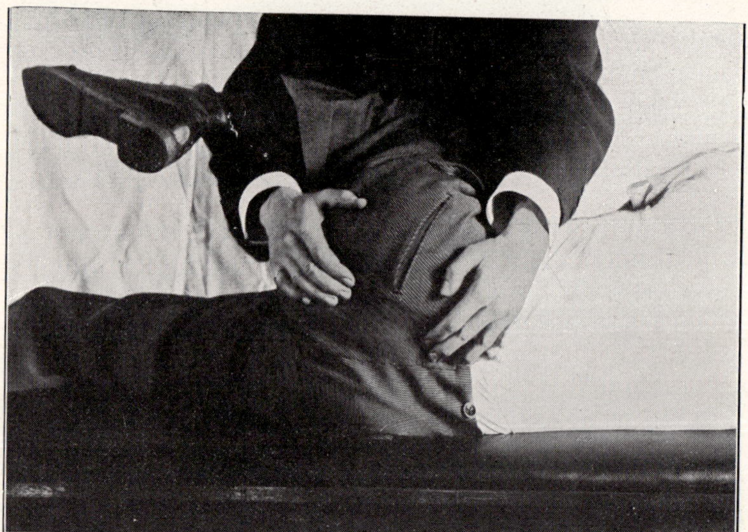

FIG. 57.—Manner of correcting a posterior innominate lesion by the wheel and axle method, also a method of taking hold of the innominate for the purpose of putting the sacro-iliac joint through its normal movements.

femur through the shaft of which, according to the angle it makes with the plane of the trunk, may be directed a force which will rotate the innominate backward and inward or outward and forward.

V. Rotation Lateral Movement.—Let B, who is assumed to have a right posterior innominate lesion, lie upon his left side on the table facing O who stands beside the table. O should flex B's left knee and place it against O's thigh to hold firmly part of the pelvis. O flexes B's right leg at the knee and places the knee against his sternum, so that B's thigh is at right angles to the plane of his trunk. O places the heel of his left hand against the anterior surface of the right tuberosity, the palm of the right hand against the posterior superior spinous process and the crest of the ilium adjacent. O now combines simultaneously a firm, unswerving pressure against B's right knee in a straight line forward, while he pushes backward on the tuberosity and pulls forward on the posterior upper part of the ilium in the effort to secure a rotation of the innominate forward and outward.

O may continue this pressure constantly for a few moments with an additional excess of force at its conclusion; he may apply the pressures with vibration for some moments, or he may repeat, with intermediate relaxation, the efforts at correction.

VI. Supine Rotation Movement.—Let B, having the same lesion as above, lie upon his back on the table, O standing to his right side, and facing the head of the table. O pulls B laterally toward him until the tuberosity of the right ischium escapes the table. He flexes B's right leg to a right angle and carrying it laterally until the femur lies in a plane parallel to the sacro-iliac articulation, he places the knee under his right axilla. O places his hands over and back of B's hip until they can exert a forward pull upon the posterior third of the crest of the right ilium. The two pressures are made coincidentally, downward and backward upon the femur, and upward and forward upon the iliac crest; thus, two points of attack are made use of in this movement.

VII. Upright Rotation Movement.—Ask B to stand with the left innominate and sacrum against a door jamb. He is instructed to flex his right knee to a right angle with his body wall. O carries the flexed knee laterally a little and rests the knee against his own left thigh or hip bone. He takes hold of the right tuberosity to push it backward while with his left hand he pulls upon the posterior third of the iliac crest to bring it forward and outward.

The principle applied in this movement is exactly the same

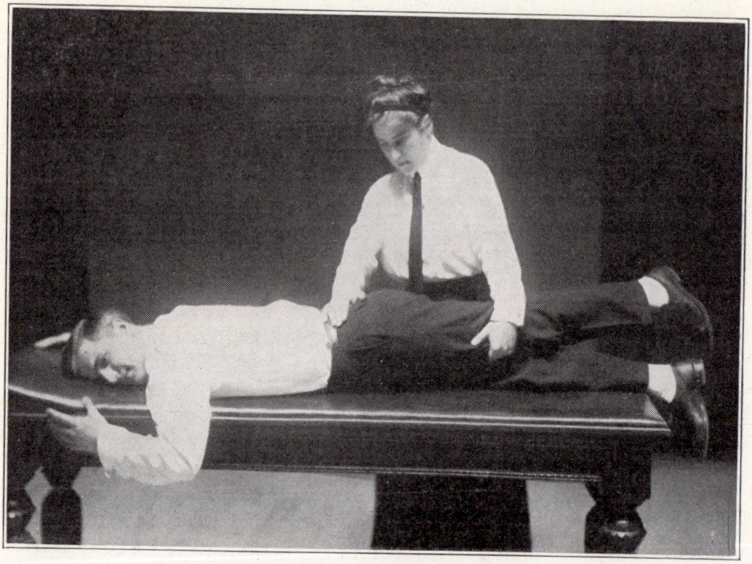

FIG. 58.—Illustrating the scissors movement for the correction of a posterior innominate lesion.

as in the rotation lateral movement save that the position of B's body is upright instead of lateral.[1]

VIII. SCISSORS' MOVEMENT.—Ask B to lie prone upon the table. O stands to his left and places his left hand upon the lower part of B's sacrum to hold it as a fixed point against which the right innominate may be rotated by a pull upon the anterior superior spine and adjacent osseous surfaces. O reaches across and lifts B's right leg by taking hold of it above the knee. He carries the thigh across the left one and with recurring tension and relaxation exerts a pull upon the innominate which is sufficient to adjust it.

The left hand may be placed against the posterior superior spine to add to the pulling of the thigh muscles described above, a thrust in a direction to push the ilium outward and forward.[2]

1. The student should plan in this manner how he may vary corrective movements by changing the patient's position. In the case of the scissors' movement, the patient might lie upon the floor, or stand against the door-jamb, facing it and the movement would be practically unvaried. It is essential to know the principles of correction and have some experience in handling the body mass of patients before it is possible to combine position and leverages in the perfection of an elaborate technique.

2. Dr. Kendall L. Achorn, in the "Jour. of the A. O. A.", June, 1913, pg. 617, (b), described a vibratory method of correcting this lesion which he uses instead of the scissors' movement. It consists in applying vibration to the posterior superior spine in the right direction for adjustment.

IX. LEG-SWINGING MOVEMENT.—Ask B to lie supine upon the table, with his right innominate projecting beyond the edge of the table. O stands to his right and reaches under with his left hand until he can grasp the tuberosity of the right ischium. He lets the posterior superior spine and the adjacent crest of the ilium rest against his left forearm. With the right hand he carries B's right leg off from the table and presses downward upon it above the knee to cause a tension in the muscles attached to the anterior superior spine and adjacent surfaces. Pulling backward and upward upon the tuberosity and iliac crest, and pushing downward and outward upon B's thigh, by repeated attempts, or by steady action with an increase in force at conclusion, the lesion may be adjusted.

X. SACRUM-LEVERAGE MOVEMENT.—Ask B to lie prone upon the table with the left leg off the table, its weight resting easily upon the toes. O stands beside the table on B's left. He places the heel of his left hand against the right posterior superior spine, his right hand against the lower part of the sacrum to assist B in its extension. B is asked to bring himself back in extension as far as possible without lifting the pelvis from the table. This may be repeated several times at one treatment.

In some cases it is better for O to place both hands over the right posterior superior spine and when B brings the sacrum back in extension, after repeated efforts making certain that the articulation has been prepared, give a direct and sudden increase of force against the ilium for adjustment. It may require thirty foot-pounds of power to overcome the lesion.

This movement without the assistance of O may be taken as an exercise for all patients who have shown any improvement in the motion of the posteriorly lesioned sacro-iliac articulation.

AFTER-TREATMENT

This is largely that of prevention of recurrence. It is undeniably true that no osseous lesion exists without atony of the stretched muscle tissues and without contracture of the shortened fasciculi. Unequal muscular tension signifies disturbed equilibrium and the lower down this loss of symmetry occurs, the more apt is it to recur through the influence of weight carriage. It is for this reason that the patients having innominate lesions should be advised to study the habits of their daily lives to find out what actions may seem to induce a recurrence or strain the joint. From knowledge of previous cases the physician should advise the patient to sit erect before turning over in bed, to avoid standing upon one foot, crossing the knees, walking with heels of unequal height, stooping to one side, and bending upon one knee.

FLEXION OF THE OS COXÆ

Flexion of the innominate is accomplished by immobilizing the os coxæ and moving the sacrum and other innominate, as one, backward in extension. If strain or infective process should cause a permanent immobilization of the articulation, an anterior innominate lesion would be produced.

EXPERIMENTAL PALPATION, M.—Ask the subject, B, to lie prone upon the table, with his left leg and innominate dropping off the edge of the table but resting the weight in ease upon the foot on the floor. With his hands palm downward upon the table, B raises himself backward in extension while O palpates the sacro-iliac articulations, comparing the motion in both joints, the measurements between the posterior superior spines and a certain

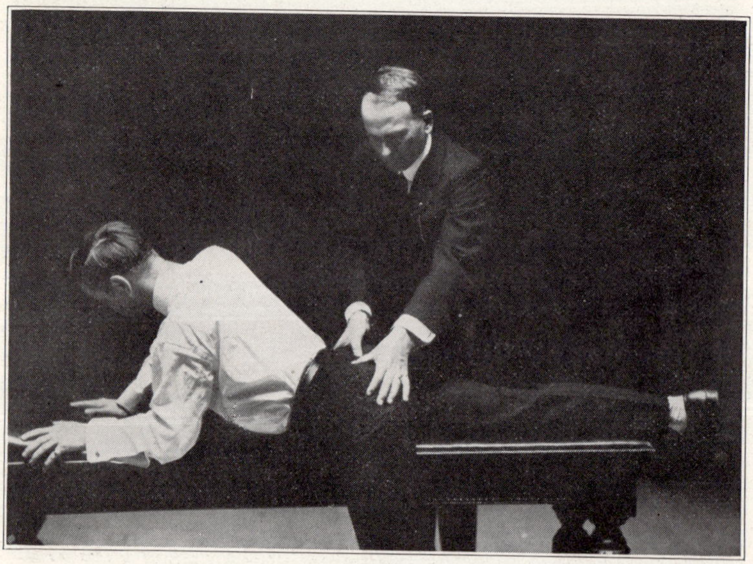

FIG. 59.—Illustrating the experimental production and palpation of an anterior innominate lesion.

point upon the sacrum, and the levels of the bony surfaces before the motion begins and at its termination. With a steel tape, while B holds the position of flexion, O verifies his conclusions arrived at by palpation, which may be summarized as follows:

The sacrum and left innominate have moved as one bone backward upon the right innominate above the axis of rotation and forward upon the innominate below the axis of motion.

The distance between the posterior superior spine of the right iluim and the spinous process of the second sacral segment is greater than the distance between the same corresponding points upon the left side.

In forward rotation of the innominate, the distance between the coccygeal extremity of the sacrum and the ischium must be lessened, causing the sacro-sciatic ligaments to become lax. The forward rotation would also depress the left side of the pubic symphysis.

The anterior innominate lesion may be defined as an immobilization of the sacro-iliac articulation in the position of extension of the sacrum or flexion of the innominate.

Its diagnosis is established by the presence of the following signs:

1. Flattening of the posterior superior spine.
2. Restricted motion in the articulation.
3. Distance between posterior superior spine and a fixed point on sacrum is less than upon the opposite side.
4. Sacro-sciatic ligaments of same side relaxed.
5. Corresponding side of os pubis depressed.

The following auxilliary signs may or may not be present:

1. Tenderness and pain upon pressure over the articulation.
2. Distance between a fixed point on the sternum and the anterior superior spines of the ilia greater on the lesioned side.
3. Measurement of the apparent length of the sides by comparing the heels, shows the heel upon the side of the lesioned innominate longer.
4. Measurement between the same fixed point on the sternum and the two malleoli shows a greater distance on the side of the lesioned innominate.

The examination of a patient having the symptoms[1] of which those afflicted with this lesion complain, should be made after the manner of examination for a posterior innominate with the differential diagnosis established by the presence of the unfailing signs.

---

1. The anterior innominate lesion is the indirect etiologic foundation for conditions which express themselves by the following symptoms: nervous disturbances, pelvic misplacements, amenorrhea, dysmenorrhea, cystitis, pain in the knee, and weakness of the ankle and foot.

CORRECTIVE MOVEMENTS

THE PRINCIPLES OF CORRECTION FOR AN ANTERIOR INNOMINATE LESION ARE EXTENSION OF THE SACRUM OR FLEXION OF THE INNOMINATE.

GENERAL RULES.—SINCE THE MOTION OF THE SACRO-ILIAC ARTICULATION IS ROTARY AND ARTHRODIAL IN CHARACTER, ALL ADJUSTIVE MOVEMENTS MUST HAVE FOR THEIR PURPOSE BACKWARD ROTATION AND INWARD GLIDING OF THE INNOMINATE.

The points of attack upon the innominate for correction of the anterior innominate lesion, are the anterior superior spine, the tuberosity of the ischium, the hamstring muscles pulling upon the ischium, and the femur in the acetabulum at an obtuse angle to the plane of the body wall.

XI. BACKWARD ROTATION MOVEMENT.—Let the patient, B, who is assumed to have an anterior innominate lesion upon the right, lie upon his left side on the table facing O who stands beside him. O flexes B's knees at obtuse angles, places the right against the upper part of his sternum, the left against his thigh to hold

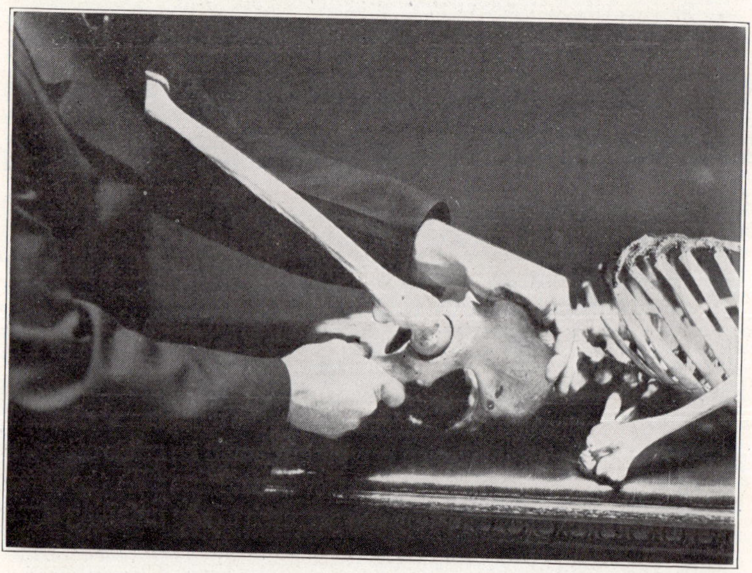

FIG. 60.—Illustrating the wheel and axle method of correction of an anterior innominate lesion, showing the angle which the femur should make with the horizontal plane of the table.

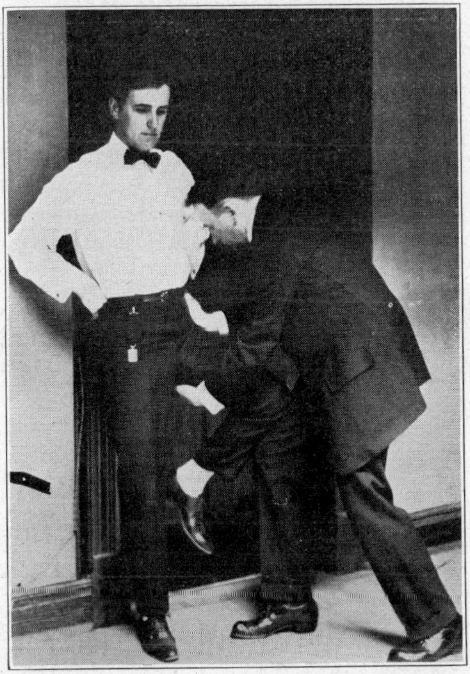

Fig. 61.—Illustrating a movement of correction for an anterior innominate lesion.

the pelvis firmly. He grasps the right ischial tuberosity to pull it forward, and places the heel of his right hand against the anterior superior spine of B's right innominate to rotate it backward. Pressure is made simultaneously against the three points of attack, each movement being in a different direction from the other two. The pressure may be increased at its conclusion, it may be given in vibratory fashion, or it may be given with alternate strong force and relaxation. Adjustment does not usually occur with any sound whatsoever, and verification of correction must be had by the absence of the diagnostic signs.

B's anterior innominate lesion may also be corrected by the same procedure when he lies upon his back on the table, with the right innominate free of the table. The knee of the right innominate is placed in O's right axilla, the thigh flexed at an obtuse angle with the plane of the trunk and the shaft of the femur abducted until it lies in a plane parallel to the articular surfaces of the right sacro-iliac joint.

XII. UPRIGHT BACKWARD ROTATION MOVEMENT.—The patient, B, is directed to stand against the door-jamb with the left innominate and the sacrum resting against the jamb as a fixed point against which to rotate the right innominate as in the above manner.

XIII. WEIGHT PULLING MOVEMENT.[1]—Ask the patient, B, to lie across the table prone, with the head and shoulder girdle hanging free upon one side, with the anterior superior iliac spines resting on the table on the opposite side, the pubes and thighs being free of the table. O stands behind and to the right of B and steps with his left foot between B's legs, placing his right hand upon the base of B's sacrum. With his left hand he grasps B's right leg at the ankle and raises it until it is at a right angle with B's thigh. O then puts his right tibia in the bend of B's knee. O lets a small amount of weight rest against B's leg to abduct it until the shaft of the femur lies in a plane parallel to the sacro-iliac joint. O then puts a considerable amount of pressure suddenly down upon B's leg to pull in backward rotation the right innominate, meanwhile holding firmly the sacrum as a fixed point.

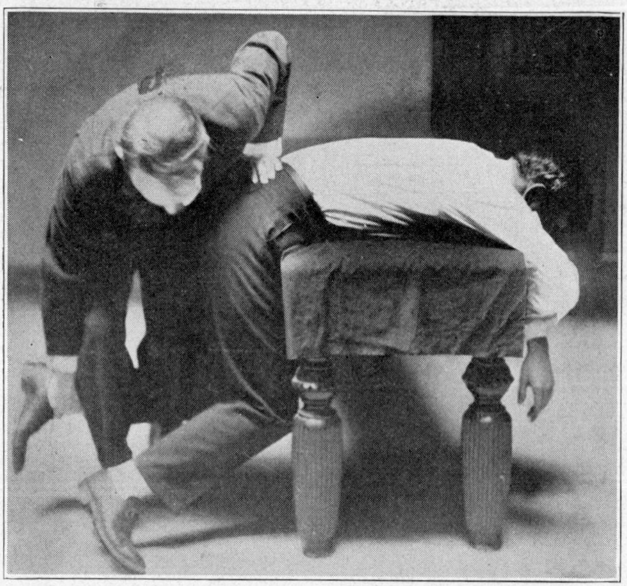

FIG, 62.—Illustrating the weight pulling method of adjusting an anterior innominate lesion.

1. This movement has been well described and illustrated by Dr. Reginald Platt of Minneapolis in current osteopathic literature.

XIV. REENFORCED FIXATION MOVEMENT.[1]—Ask the patient B, to lie upon his left side upon the table and carry the shoulders prone upon the table by dropping the left arm off from the table behind him. This extreme rotation of the trunk is for the purpose of adding a secondary fixation of the sacrum by the pull of the lumbosacral and ilio-lumbar ligaments of the right side.

O stands behind B and places his right knee against the base of B's sacrum to make of it a fixed point. O then reaches over B and takes hold of his right leg at the knee, flexes it at an obtuse angle with the plane of the body wall, and puts a great deal of strength into pulling backward upon the knee while raising it upward from the table and outward from the mesial plane of the body. O may place his left hand or his lateral thoracic wall against B's back to assist in maintaining the fixation of the sacrum against which the innominate is rotated.

The movement should not be repeated more than twice at a treatment for it is one of exceedingly great force and should be used with caution.

XV. SACRAL FLEXION MOVEMENT.—Let B sit upon the table with his right leg outstretched, the left leg dropped off the side of the table and the left innominate clear of the table at the ischial tuberosity. O stands to the left of B and places his right hand upon B's lower thoracic area, his left hand across B's thigh just above the knee. Under B's right heel a brick of four to six inches may be placed to raise the heel and to increase the pull of the hamstring muscles upon that side.

O bends B forward in flexion to move the sacrum and other innominate as one upon the innominate in lesion. The correction obtained by this means is usually gradual. The movement may be given following adjustment to exaggerate the lesion slightly for the purpose of over-correction, a method which helps to stretch contracted tissues.

Patients may make an exercise of the movement for home use, to keep the ligaments of the articulation pliable between treatments.

The patient with an anterior innominate lesion should be warned that certain movements predispose to a recurrence of the lesion and aggravate the case before adjustment has been secured.

---

1. This movement is not recommended for the use of the undergraduate. Its leverage is very powerful and it should be used only after other methods have failed. The graduate osteopath who has acquired skill in palpation so that he is able to detect the moment that movement begins in an articulation under correction is qualified to use the movement intelligently.

Going down an inclined plane as down hill, down many flights of stairs, stepping from the high car steps of street cars with the foot of the afflicted side in advance, jumping which brings a strain upon both joints and more effectively upon the lesioned one, prolonged sitting in a backward slumped position which causes an extension of the sacrum, all are to be avoided as much as possible before adjustment is complete and muscular equilibrium has been attained.

Two classes of lesions occur in the sacro-iliac articulation, impaction and relaxation lesions.[1] The impaction lesion is difficult or impossible of adjustment for when a thinning of the cartilaginous tissues takes place in the joint there are usually irritative changes going on which result in exostoses and fibrous ankylosis. If the vibratory method will not loosen the articulation so that the physician or the patient can detect a slight degree of mobility after a few weeks' trial, it is probably a joint that is past help. A number of such specimens, seen at Wistar Institute, Philadelphia, a part of the excellent osteological collection in that institution, would prove to the student that many people are afflicted with impaction lesions of one or both sacro-iliac joints.

The hypermobile sacro-iliac articulation usually accompanies a lesion of the opposite side characterized by more or less fixation. Examination should be made of the other joint to ascertain if its motion is sufficient; if it is not, treatment should be given it to increase its mobility. At the same time exercises for the general strengthening and equilibration of the spinal muscles should be advised, these exercises to consist in movements of flexion and extension which shall dvelop the muscles of both sides of the back at the same time. A method which may be called the irritative method, is often employed to assist in fixing the innominate. It consists in a forcible jarring of the bony surfaces adjacent to the articulation. The hand is placed palm downward, either upon the outer surface of the ilium adjacent to the posterior superior spinous process or upon the sacrum just internal to the ilium, and then the other hand doubled in a fist, strikes the dorsal surface of the hand in position against the joint several blows as hard as the hand can

---

1. See page 10, last paragraph, and page 11, first paragraph.

bear. This will set up in the joint an irritation sufficient to shorten the relaxed ligaments.

Recurrent innominate lesions, which simulate the hypermobile articulation, are treated in much the same way, following adjustment of the lesion. These cases should be over-corrected before the irritative procedure is begun.

The physician should not overlook the possibility of lumbar lesions accompanying sacro-iliac lesions and offering an etiologic basis for failure in adjustment. Lesions of the fourth and fifth lumbar articulations are the most common lesions and are either primary or secondary, and should be corrected.

Counterbalancing lesions occur early in the case following an innominate lesion. They may be lateral lumbar lesions, a functional curvature usually of the lumbar area, or a secondary lesion of the other innominate, of the opposite type.

SACROCOCCYGEAL LESIONS

The joint made by the sacrum and coccyx[1] is of the nature of a symphysis with an interarticular cartilage between the two bones. The ligaments of the articulation are strong but pliable allowing some movement in the joint normally in the direction of flexion and extension. The upward and forward pull of the levator ani muscle prevents extreme backward extension.

The lesions of this joint are usually the result of traumatism or parturition. There are flexion, extension, rotation, and lateral bending lesions found in this joint.

Examination is made per rectum for the purpose of diagnosis. The normal articulation shows a fair amount of motion in the direction of extension and flexion. When lesion is present, motion is restricted or lost; more or less tenderness is present upon palpation of the adjacent osseous margins of the bones in the articulation. The patient usually gives a history of strain by traumatism or in delivery.

A lesion may be differentiated from dislocation-fracture of the coccyx, a fairly common disturbance, by absence of crepitus, abnormal mobility, and great pain about the joint.

1. See Morris, ibid., page 238, ninth paragraph.

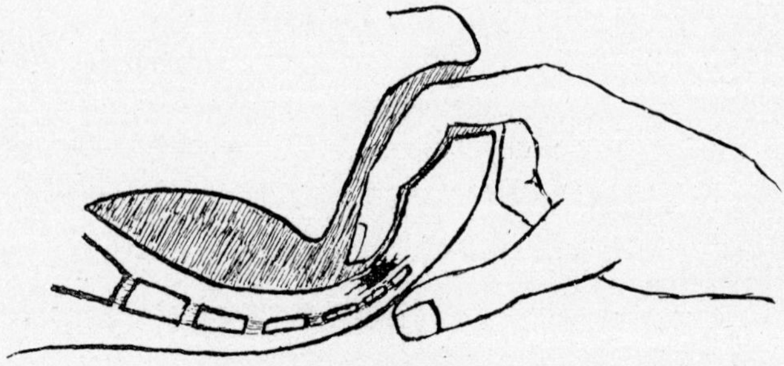

FIG. 63—Drawing to illustrate the manner of grasping the coccyx per rectum for adjustment of sacrococcygeal lesions.

Coccygeal lesion or dislocation makes difficult rising or sitting in chairs, defecation, and forward bending.

An extension lesion of the coccyx is one in which the sacrococcygeal articulation is immobilized in the position of backward bending. The principle of its correction is forward flexion, accomplished by grasping the coccyx between the thumb on its posterior surface and the index finger on its anterior surface through the rectum, and after stretching the tissues about the joint by attempting to put it through its normal movements, with a slight downward traction and with flexion forward, it is adjusted. Often the condition is one of ankylosis and surgical removal is indicated.

An anterior coccyx is one which is immobilized in the position of flexion. Its principle of correction is extension.

A rotated coccyx is a lesion in which the coccyx is maintained in the position of rotation on a vertical axis, the rotation being to the right or to the left with additional flexion. Its correction consists in retracing the path taken in its displacement and is accomplished by the manner offered above of grasping the coccyx and replacing it. Treatment of the sacro-sciatic ligaments is valuable in preparation for the adjustment.

A lateral coccyx is one which is usually the result of direct violence or it may be associated with structural curvature of the spine. It is a lesion in which the coccyx is immobilized in a position of lateral gliding upon the sacrum. Its correction may be attempted after the manner of the adjustment of the other lesions of this joint and will be successful if ankylosis has not occurred.

PELVIC INCLINATION

For two purposes is consideration given to the subject of pelvic inclination, the first for the important bearing it has upon the delivery of the child and secondly in reference to the posture of the body as a foundation for lateral curvature, scoliosis, and group lesions.

Pelvic inclination is a term which is used to designate the relation which the pelvis bears to the horizon. The line by which it is determined is a line which is projected from the lumbosacral angle to the upper border of the symphysis pubis and the angle that line makes with the horizon is spoken of as the angle of inclination. It may be readily seen that if the back part of the pelvis is elevated or the front part lowered, the angle of inclination is increased; if the back part is lowered or the pubes elevated, the angle of inclination is diminished. That part of the line which extends from the lumbosacral angle to the symphysis pubis is called the conjugate vera or internal conjugate diameter and its measurement is important when consideration of the pelvic inlet as a whole is to be determined in the study of the case of the expectant mother.

Other measurements taken by obstetricians are: (a) between the iliac crests; (b) between the anterior superior spines; (c) between the posterior superior spines; (d) between the tuber ischii; (e) between the iliac crests; (f) between the tip of the coccyx and the under edge of the symphysis. When a comparison is made between the figures given in any authoritative medical text upon the subject of obstetrics, with the figures which are suggested in this book in reference to changes wrought in sacral flexion and sacral extension, the deduction is logically made that the cause of the difference lies in the relation of the sacrum to the two innominates. Researches have been undertaken by some of the cleverest investigators of the other schools of practice, among whom may be mentioned Prochovnik,[1] Henggeler,[2] Engelhard,[3] Robert W. Lovett,[4] Joel Goldthwait,[5] but not one of them has

1. "Archib. f. Gyn." 1882, XIX, I. 2. "Zeitsch, f. orth. Chir.", XII, 4, 613. 3. "Zeitsch. f. ortho. Chir." XXVII, p. 1, 1910. 4. Ibidem, p. 17-19.
5. Bos. Med. and Surg. Jour., June 17, 1915. He recognizes "strain" of the sacro-iliac joint but not subluxation in the sense of immobilization or, as osteopathists term it, lesion.

been able to understand the fundamental reason for the differences. Lovett very honestly states that the whole subject of pelvic inclination must be left in an unsatisfactory and unsettled condition[1] and it is by reason of the failure of all investigators to recognize the bilateral sacro-iliac lesion.

A review of the findings[2] in sacral lesion may be stated in the terms of obstetric measurements, thus:

A. In sacral flexion lesions, the angle of pelvic inclination is greater and the distance between the

1. Sacral promontory and symphysis or the conjugate vera is decreased.
2. Anterior superior spines less.
3. Posterior superior spines less.
4. Coccyx and under edge of symphysis pubis greater.
5. Tuber ischii greater.

B. In sacral extension lesions, the angle of pelvic inclination is less and the distance between the

1. Sacral promontory and the symphysis pubis is greater.
2. Anterior superior spines greater.
3. Posterior superior spines greater.
4. Coccyx and under edge of the symphysis pubis less.
5. Tuber ischii less.

Sacral flexion lesions are followed by lordosis of the lumbar area, kyphosis of the dorsal area, and round shoulders. The degree of lesion varies, therefore the sequelæ vary, but the main difference between the normal pelvis and that having the sacral flexion lesion may be found in the presence of the signs stated above.

Sacral extension lesions are followed by the straight spine and the flat chest when the lesion is extreme. That great variance exists in the degrees of lesion may be readily perceived when we remember that Prochovnik states that he found the average of his collected results showed the variation in males in pelvic inclination to be from 44 to 60 degrees, in women from 41 to 65 degrees. The pertinent question is, who has normal[3] sacro-iliac articulations?

1. His own words, loc. cit.
2. Pages 131 and 134.
3. It is the author's opinion that at the present time only palpation of the most skilled physician can determine the answer.

CHAPTER VIII

RIB LESIONS

A rib lesion is a subluxation or an immobilization of a rib in a position of normal respiratory movement. It usually results from an incomplete inspiration or expiration. Occasionally it may be due to a restriction which holds the rib from taking part in normal movements. As the result of direct violence, fracture, not subluxation, is produced. Rare instances of dislocations of the first and twelfth ribs have been reported but with these we are not concerned.

A true rib lesion is independent of any spinal lesion; it is present on one side of a vertebra only, and it must not be confounded with the changed positions of the ribs attached to a vertebra that has become immobilized in lesion. A rib in articulation with a lesioned vertebra is not itself immobilized; its range of movement may be less than the normal; it may show a slight elevation at the angle and a depression at the chondral extremity, or the reverse, but differential diagnosis will reveal the presence of a lesion of the vertebra with which it articulates doubly and treatment will be directed toward the correction of the spinal lesion, frequently with the assistance of rib leverage.

For mechanical purposes, the ribs may be divided into four classes:

1. The first rib.
2. The ribs from the second to the sixth inclusive.
3. The seventh, eight, ninth, and tenth ribs.
4. The eleventh and twelfth ribs.

The ribs of the first three classes have two articulations with the vertebræ corresponding in number; each of the second and third classes of ribs articulates also with the vertebra above; the first rib sometimes articulates with the body of the seventh cervical; the eleventh and twelfth ribs articulate with the bodies only of the corresponding thoracic vertebræ and are properly called "floating ribs."

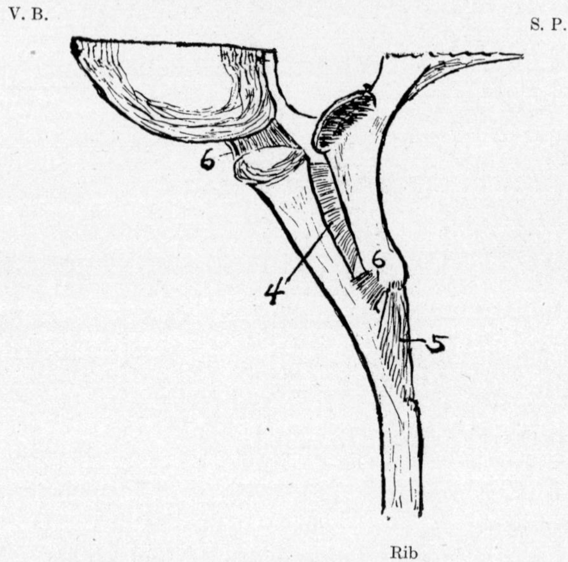

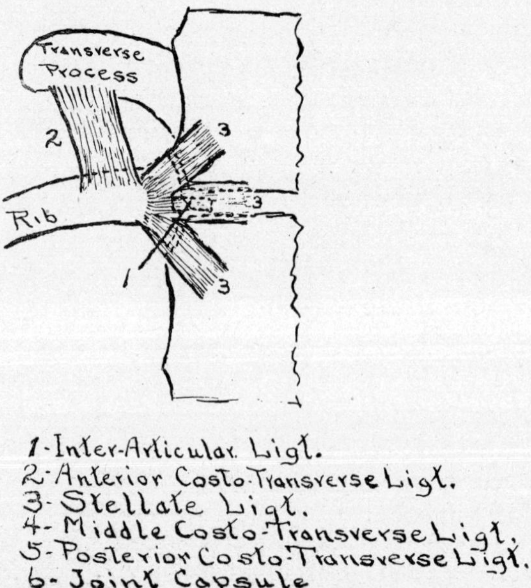

FIGS. 64 AND 65—Drawings to illustrate the connection of a rib with the vertebræ. Additional figures: V.B., body of vertebræ; S.P., spinous process.

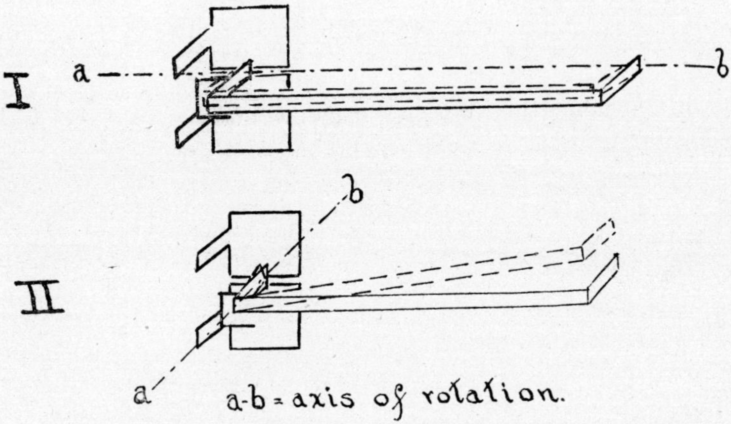

FIG. 66—Drawings to illustrate the movements of the ribs in respiration: (I) upon a sterno-vertebral axis and (II) upon a costotransverse axis, the first axis being that which characterizes movement of the seventh to tenth ribs inclusive, only; the second axis being that of the second to the tenth ribs inclusive.

The articulations of a typical rib, for an example the right third rib, are:

1. A costocentral joint, formed by the head of the third rib and the cavities on the contiguous surfaces of the second and third thoracic vertebral bodies and the intervertebral disc between them. Its character is that of an arthrodial joint.

2. A costotransverse joint formed by the articular surfaces on the tubercle of the rib and the adjacent transverse process. It is also arthrodial in type.

3. Anteriorly through its cartilage, with which it is almost inseparably united, it forms with the sternum a ginglymus joint.

The axis of its motion[1] corresponds with a line drawn through the two articulations with the vertebra, by means of which the rib, as it rotates slightly downward posteriorly and glides as in an arc on the transverse process of the vertebra, turns upward in front and moves forward as though to thrust the sternum anterior. This is the movement of the second class of ribs in inspiration and may be the first part of the inspiratory movement of the third division of ribs.

1. See: Cunningham, ibid, p. 317, paragraph 6.
Gray, ibid., p. 285, under heading "Movements."

In expiration, the antero-posterior diameter of the thorax decreases, the rib glides upward at its costotransverse articulation, rotates upward at its costocentral joint, and is depressed anteriorly. Forced respiratory movements will with the aid of careful palpation prove these movements of the ribs.

An **inspiration lesion**[1] of one of the second division of ribs is a subluxation or immobilization of that rib in the position of forced inspiration; it is elevated at its anterior extremity and depressed at its angle.

The diagnosis of such a lesion is established by the presence of the following invariable signs:

1. Immobility of the rib in respiratory movement.
2. Elevation of the anterior or chondral extremity of the rib with some eversion of the lower border of its shaft.
3. Depression of the angle of the rib, with approximation to the one below.

Patients who have rib lesions usually complain of a pain located between two ribs, in the anterior axillary line, close to the angle of the rib, or nearer to the spine in the region of the transverse process. The pain is a localized one, sharp in character, nearly always constantly present, and mitigated only by application of counter-irritants. Careful physical diagnosis can reveal no organic cause for the pain. It remains for its etiology to be established by finding a rib lesion present.

Examination should be made of the whole outer surface of the rib from its junction with the transverse process to its chondral articulation. This shall be done by palpation, if possible upon the skin; if not, because of the exposure of the person, through a very thin, soft texture. Palpation must be carefully made, with warm hands, with light pressure, and by varying the position of the patient and the shoulder girdle. The vertebræ in articulation with the rib should be examined first of all for lesions. It is possible, however, for a rib lesion and a vertebral lesion to be present at one and the same time.

The relation of the rib in question to the one above and the one below should be noted throughout its length. With the palm

1. This lesion has been called in osteopathic literature "a rib that is down in the back and up in front."

of the hand laid against the rib, with the fingers resting between its borders and those of the adjoining ribs, the patient should be asked to take a full inspiration and then give a complete expiration. By this test for motion, it may be determined whether or not a lesion exists. The physician may stand behind the patient, who is spare enough to show the ribs in respiratory movements, clasp his hands in front below the patient's sixth ribs and compress firmly his chest wall so that he shall limit movement to the upper ribs. If lesion is present, the physician will note, by scanning the anterior chest wall, whether or not there is any failure of a rib to take part in the movement. If all rise equally, lesion is not present and the symptoms are probably due to a vertebral lesion.

CORRECTIVE MOVEMENTS

THE PRINCIPLE OF CORRECTION FOR AN INSPIRATION RIB LESION IS UPWARD AND BACKWARD ROTATION AT THE VERTEBRAL EXTREMITY OF THE RIB.

GENERAL RULES.—SINCE THE RIBS HAVE SOME ELASTICITY IN THEIR STRUCTURE, COMPRESSION OF THE EXTREMITIES OF THE RIBS MAY BE USED IN ASSISTING TO ADJUST THEM. DISENGAGEMENT OF THE COSTOTRANSVERSE ARTICULATION MAY BE OBTAINED IN THIS WAY.

When one takes into consideration the small axis of motion upon which the rib turns, it may be easily seen that no adjustment can be successful that is coarse and large. The range of movement in each of the joints, the costotransverse and costocentral, is limited. Although anteriorly the separation between the chondral extremity and that of the rib below seems very noticeable, it is due to the fact that the cartilaginous articulation is at the end of the radius while the angle is near the centre of motion, the costocentral joint, and the difference in the amount of movement of these two must necessarily be great.

No treatment need cause pain. The confidence of the patient is most easily shaken by rough technique.[1] The points of attack

1. Great deftness is required in the correction of these lesions. The tissues about the ribs, especially the mammary glands, may be seriously injured by rough work, and no physician should be excused who attempts a coarse, heavy movement for the adjustment of an articulation as small in extent of its articulating surfaces as the costotransverse.

of avail are the angle and the anterior extremity of the rib. Respiratory movement may assist; inspiration lesions will best be adjusted at the conclusion of or during expiration when there is relaxation of the muscles that assist in elevating the thorax.

I. PRONE ANGLE MOVEMENT.—The patient, B, is assumed to have an inspiration lesion of the right third rib. He is asked to lie prone with his arms hanging over the end of the table. O stands to his left and places the left hand underneath B, down over his chest until he rests the palmer surfaces of the middle and index fingers against the upper border of the lesioned rib. The heel of O's right hand is placed under the angle of the rib behind or he may use here the palmar surface of his right thumb or his elbow, as is most suitable to him. B is asked to make the cycle of a full inspiration and then an expiration, and at the close of expiration O puts a sudden firm pressure against the angle of the rib to raise it upward, and against the other extremity to carry it downward, which, if the tension is just right, will result in correction.

This movement will adjust any rib in inspiration lesion from the second to the ninth. It may be varied by having the patient lie upon the back, O standing to B's left and reaching between the shoulders to pull with the finger-tips the angle upward while with the heel of the hand the rib is pushed downward anteriorly.

II. A. T. S. CHAIR MOVEMENT.—Let B, the patient, be assumed to have an inspiration lesion of the right sixth rib. He is asked to sit upon a chair that has a high straight back or upon a chair especially arranged for the correction of rib lesions[1], with his left side against the back of the chair, to support and immobilize the left side of the thorax so that no movement made for correction of the lesion will cause any movement in the other side. O stands to the right of B and raising B's right arm places it over his shoulder.

O places the thumb of his left hand under the angle of B's sixth rib, the fingers of his right hand over the same rib anteriorly. During one of B's expirations, O raises the angle of the rib posteriorly, pushes it down anteriorly, to adjust the lesion. It may require compression of the extremities of the rib to disengage the costotransverse articulation before adjustment can be successfully accomplished.

This movement will correct an inspiration lesion of any rib from the fourth to the ninth.

---

1. Dr. A. T. Still has devised a chair for this express purpose. It has an upright curved piece of galvanized iron supported by two rods, which with a pillow under the axilla of the patient makes an excellent support.

III. ELBOW COMPRESSION MOVEMENT.[1]—Let B, the patient, be assumed to have an inspiration lesion of the right fifth rib. B is asked to lie supine upon the table without a pillow to support his head. O places the fingers of his left hand under the scapula until they reach the angle of the rib which is down. They grasp this angle with the purpose of raising it; or, if O prefers, he can place a knuckle under the angle of the rib to offer pressure and resistance at the moment of correction.

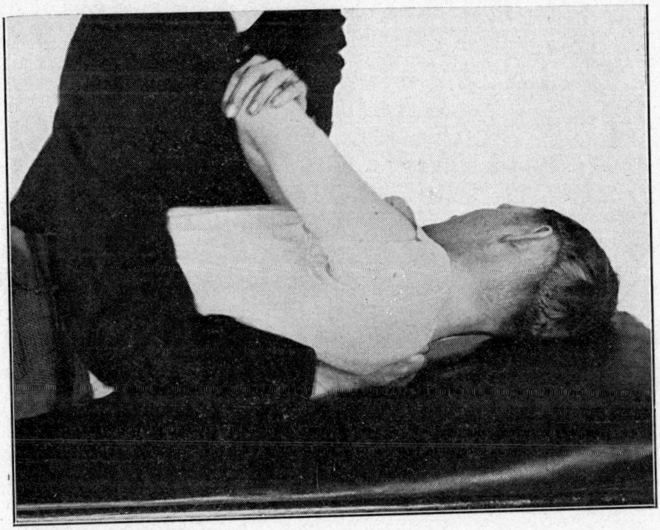

FIG. 67—Illustrating the elbow compression movement for the correction of an inspiration lesion of the left fourth rib.

O then grasps B's right elbow and moves it transversely across his chest so that it lies over the anterior extremity of the rib in lesion. With his hand upon the right elbow, O tries the range of movement that is required to bring a pull through the muscles upon the fifth rib and also to test the point at which compression[2]

1. The author has observed that osteopaths differ in what they consider the best position of the patient for the adjustment of rib lesions. Dr. Still and his sons seem to prefer to have the patient seated upon a stool; Dr. Frank Farmer with them seated upon the side of a table in front of him; Dr. H. W. Forbes, the patient lying prone or supine upon the table, working usually upon the posterior extremity of the rib.

2. No extremely forcible compression should be used to assist in correcting rib lesions for in many people ribs are brittle and may fracture easily, especially is this true of the ribs from the sixth to the eighth. Rib lesions are not as frequently found as was formerly supposed and when found care should be used in the choice of osteopathic operative measures.

is most successful in moving the rib. With his two hands working in conjunction O may easily adjust the lesion.

This movement will adjust any inspiration rib lesion from the fourth to the eighth ribs, inclusive. The above movements may be varied by position according to the habit of the physician and the weight of the patient. Inspiration lesions are less common than those of the other classes and types.

An **expiration lesion**[1] is one in which any rib from the second to the tenth inclusive is maintained in a position of forced or exaggerated expiration; it is depressed at its anterior extremity and elevated at its angle. Its diagnosis is established by the presence of the following signs:

1. Immobility of the rib in respiratory movement.
2. Depression of the chondral extremity of the rib with some eversion of its upper border and with approximation to the rib below.
3. Elevation of the angle of the rib posteriorly with prominence of its lower border and separation from the angle of the rib below.

The expiration lesion is the commonest of the rib lesions. It is usually the result of accident by compression at a moment of forcible inspiration or by sharp changes[2] in the respiratory cycle not calling into use the entire thoracic capacity. The expiration lesion is not difficult of adjustment for its angle, prominent often in the plane of the back and always to touch, offers an excellent point of attack.

CORRECTIVE MOVEMENTS

THE PRINCIPLE OF CORRECTION FOR AN EXPIRATION LESION IS DOWNWARD AND BACKWARD ROTATION AT THE VERTEBRAL EXTREMITY OF THE RIB.

---

1. This lesion has been called "a rib up in the back and down in front."

2. As an example of this class of cases one may be cited in point: a young woman in playing tennis jumped to strike a ball and missed it. Her arm had gathered momentum carrying it beyond voluntary control and her racket struck her ankle. The cycle of respiratory events was first a sudden expiration instantaneously following the missed stroke. Then a sharp inspiratory movement in an effort to regain control of the arm, synchronously with which she was seized with a stinging pain somewhere among the ribs under her arm. It was due to a failure on the part of the seventh rib to take part in the sudden movement of inspiration. Examination years afterward for the cause of the pain which had never ceased, revealed an expiration lesion of the right seventh rib. (Patient examined in consultation with Dr. Wm. Gardner of Rockford, Ill.)

GENERAL RULE.—EXPIRATION LESIONS MAY BE CORRECTED BEST AT THE MOMENT OF FULL INSPIRATION.

IV. HYPEREXTENSION MOVEMENT.—Let the patient, B, who is assumed to have an expiration lesion of the left fifth rib, be asked to sit upon the side of a table and well back so that he may rest his right shoulder against O's right shoulder. O reaches around B with his right arm until the fingers of the right hand grasp the fifth rib anteriorly to lift it. O's left thumb, or the heel of the hand, is placed against the angle of the fifth rib to thrust it downward when at the conclusion of a full inspiration B seems to be relaxed.

V. PRONE EXTENSION MOVEMENT.—Let the patient, B, having an expiration lesion of the right fifth rib, is asked to lie prone upon the table. O stands at the left of B. O lifts B's body in some extension, usually by placing his flexed knee under B's chest. O reaches under B to reenforce the upward pressure against the anterior end of the fifth rib, while with the heel of his other hand as close to the vertebral articulation with the rib as it is possible to get, he exerts a gentle thrust forward for the purpose of disengaging the costotransverse articulation. O then grasps the lower border of the rib anteriorly to pull it up and turns the heel of the hand so that he may exert a strong pressure against the angle, in a direction forward and downward toward B's feet. At the limit of inspiration, the two pressures are made synchronously with correction of the lesion.

VI. ARM ASSISTING MOVEMENT.—Let the patient, B, lie upon his left side with the lesioned sixth rib uppermost. O stands in front of B and an assistant, C, stands behind B and grasps the elbow of B's right arm to carry it upward according to O's instructions. O places the heel of his left hand[1] strongly against the angle of the right sixth rib. O's right fingers reach under the lower border of the anterior end of the rib to pull it up. B is asked to take a full inspiration and just at the point of beginning expiration C is told to carry B's right elbow upward, outward and backward while O gives a slight thrust against the angle of the rib guiding it into place by the fingers anteriorly.

VII. HOOP-ROLLING RIB MOVEMENT.—Let the patient, B, who is assumed to have an expiration lesion of the right eighth rib, lie upon the right side. O standing in front of B holds the

1. There has been a habit with a number of osteopathic physicians of using the knee to hold the vertebral extremity of the rib fixed. In the employment of one who possesses rare skill, such a force might be permissible but it is a method more noted for its abuse than for its safe use. No student should employ it in early days of practice.

lower border of the eighth rib anteriorly with the fingers of the left hand. B is asked to put the right limb behind the left. O rests his right elbow on B's left hip, the fingers of his left hand pulling down firmly on the angle of the lesioned rib. O's left shoulder rests against B's left shoulder anteriorly and O rolls B backward slightly as at the close of an inspiration he adjusts the lesion.

This movement may be used for the correction of an expiration lesion of any of the third division of ribs. Other movements, with the patient seated on a chair as in movement II, or with the patient lying supine, may be quite easily planned and executed, having the principle of correction constantly as a foundation.

In expiration lesions of the **second rib** assistance may be given by muscular leverage.

VIII. PECTORALIS MOVEMENT.—Let the patient, B, who has an expiration lesion of the right second rib, sit upon a high stool while O stands beside him on his right. O places his left shoulder under B's right axilla with the purpose of moving it backward at the right moment. O places his right thumb under the lower border of the second rib anteriorly, his left thumb or index finger knuckle against the angle of the rib posteriorly. B is asked to take a full breath, at the conclusion of which O deftly combines the two pressures with the lifting of the shoulder and adjusts the lesion.

The same movement may be given with the patient lying supine without a pillow. O rests B's arm on his own forearm, his hand being directed to the downward movement of the rib at its angle.

Inspiration lesions of the second rib may be adjusted with the patient in the same positions as above, the arm of the patient resting over the shoulder or arm of the physician merely to hold the scapular muscles relaxed.

LESIONS OF THE FIRST RIB

The first rib differs in shape from the other ribs, is controlled by a different set of muscles and does not behave in inspiration and expiration like any of the others. The movement of the first rib is upon an antero-posterior axis. In inspiration the scaleni muscles contract and raise the rib, fixing it so that the intercostal muscles below may raise all of the other ribs to increase the diameters of the thorax. The first rib articulates on each side with the first thoracic vertebra without an interarticular ligament, hence it may glide up or down very easily at that end. Anteriorly it is closely anchored to the cartilage which is united with the sternum. Movement is more pronounced in the posterior half of the rib to which the muscles are attached.

There are no lesions of the first rib of the true inspiration and expiration type. They are rather called upward and downward subluxations. An upward lesion is the result of a sudden contraction of the scaleni muscles from a various number of causes: first, a protective contraction in an attempt to ward off a blow directed to the head; secondly, from carrying heavy weights on the shoulder with the head bent to one side to get it out of the way and the shoulder girdle fixed in a position of support by the contraction above mentioned; thirdly, from prolonged contraction due to exposure, cold; fourthly, by falls upon the head or shoulders. Downward lesions of the first rib are usually due to a failure of the muscles to contract when a demand is made upon them or when by fatigue from over-exertion they lose their tone and unbalance results with the gradual production of lesion. Depressed lesions of the first rib are rare. Upward subluxations[1] occur occasionally.

The diagnosis of a first rib lesion depends upon these signs:

1. Restricted movement upon forcible inspiration.
2. Fullness or depression at the side of the neck where the shaft of the rib passes in front of the trapezius muscle.

Differential diagnosis must be made from a rotation lesion of either the first or second thoracic vertebra. A rotation lesion turns backward the rib on the side opposite to that toward which the spinous process points. There is a slight upward turning of the first rib but it does not have restricted motion. Vertebral lesions must be corrected before adjustment of the rib lesion is attempted. The neck should be examined for the presence of cervical lesions which may have been etiologic in the production of the rib lesion, for the scaleni muscles are supplied by branches from the lower four or five cervical nerves.

---

1. The commoner symptoms of which these patients complain are pain over the shoulder, hacking cough, eczema of the hands and arms, bronchitis, functional heart disturbances, goitre, and congestive headaches. When we remember with what important structures the first rib is in relation, it is not to be doubted that it proves the irritative source of many symptoms.

EXPERIMENTAL PALPATION, N.—With the subject, B, seated upon a stool with O standing behind him, O places perpendicularly to the anterior extremities of B's first ribs close to the cartilages two matches on end. B is asked to take a full breath. If there is no lesion present, the matches will be pushed upward equally. If one match does not move, that rib is in lesion.

O should carefully scan the relative height of the two shoulders at about the nape of the neck. If one is higher than the other, he should then push aside the trapezius upon that side and palpate the two first ribs to note whether or not one has greater obliquity than the other. Then with his hands applied to the upper surface of the rib, B should be asked to breathe fully. The rib which does not respond to movement is the one in lesion.

O may make a further test for motion. Placing his hand upon the top of B's head he may bend B's head to the side directly which will lift the rib by the direct pull on the muscle fibres. If the rib does not lift in this manner, lesion of the upward type is present.

CORRECTIVE MOVEMENTS

THE PRINCIPLE OF CORRECTION FOR AN UPWARD SUBLUXATION OF THE FIRST RIB IS DOWNWARD ROTATION ON THE ANTERO-

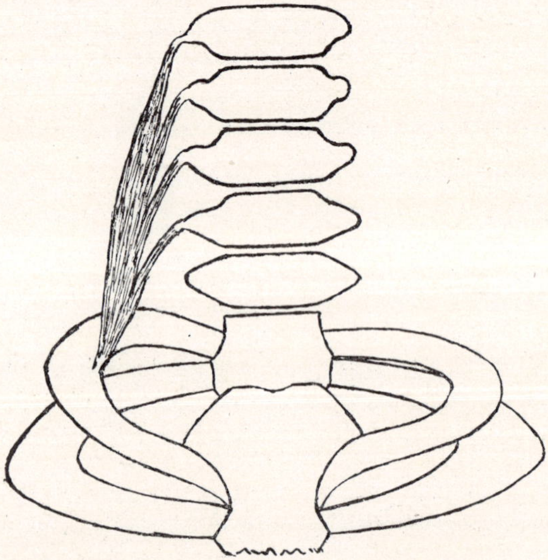

FIG. 68—Schematic drawing to illustrate the attachments of the scalenus anticus muscle and the state of contraction of that muscle in an upward subluxation of the right first rib.

POSTERIOR AXIS OF MOTION; FOR A DOWNWARD SUBLUXATION, IS UPWARD ROTATION.

GENERAL RULES.—SINCE THE UPWARD LESION HAS BEEN CAUSED BY CONTRACTION OF THE SCALENI, THESE MUSCLES MUST BE PLACED IN RELAXATION BY POSITION AND DIRECT PRESSURE USED FOR CORRECTION. IN DOWNWARD SUBLUXATION THE MUSCLES SHOULD BE USED TO LIFT THE RIB BY DIRECT PULL ALONG THEIR MUSCLE FIBRES WITH PRESSURE AGAINST THE LOWER BORDER OF THE POSTERIOR PART OF THE RIB TO ASSIST IN RAISING IT.

IX. HALF-ROTATION MOVEMENT.—Let the patient, B, who is assumed to have an upward lesion of the right first rib, sit upon a stool, O standing behind him. O places his hand upon the top of B's head, the radial side of his right index finger along the posterior third of the first rib to push it downward and slightly backward and outward at the movement of adjustment. O bends B's head to the left and then makes a quarter circumduction to the front; at this point the scaleni of both sides should be perfectly relaxed and it is then that the pressure upon the rib may adjust the lesion. If not, the head may be circumducted ninety degrees more to the right shoulder, when the right scaleni will be shortened as well as relaxed, and adjustment may be made.

X. PATIENT ASSISTING MOVEMENT.—With patient and physician seated as above, instruct the patient to perform the same movement with his head that O carried it through in the half-rotation movement. O puts his right arm under B's right axilla and raises the shoulder girdle in upward and backward circumduction to exert a pull upon the anterior end of the rib through the subclavius muscle which takes origin from the first rib and is inserted into the clavicle. Adjustment is made by the pressure downward upon the rib posteriorly as above.

XI. HEAD SIDE-BENDING MOVEMENT.—The patient, B, is assumed to have a depressed lesion of the right first rib. B and O have the same relative positions as in the above movements. O places his right thumb beneath the angle of the first rib to pry it up. O bends B's head to the opposite shoulder until tension upon the muscle is felt, then with an increase of lateral movement the rib may be raised. It should be held immobilized in the normal position while the head is circumducted to the right and through several movements of flexion and extension of the head and neck, followed by resistance on the part of the patient when flexion is attempted for the purpose of helping the scaleni to contract and return to their normal condition of tone.

Failure to adjust first rib lesions is due to the fact that they have been in existence for many years and the contractions and proliferation of connective tissue about the vertebral articulations of the rib are constrictive past the possibility of overcoming save by a long course of preliminary treatment directed to the establishment of motion in the joints. If vertebral lesions remain, it is useless to attempt to correct a rib lesion. Removal of the primary cause must always be the central thought in osteopathic procedure.

LESIONS OF THE THIRD GROUP OF RIBS

In addition to the movement which is normal to the second group of ribs, the third class has a secondary motion upon an antero-posterior axis with the object of elevating the middle part of the rib thus increasing the transverse diameter of the thorax. When these ribs are raised as in full inspiration, the lateral part is thrust outward and from its manner of action it has been compared to a bucket handle movement[1]. These lesions are probably due to direct trauma, as by lateral interference,[2] or are sequent upon vertebral lesions. They are called inspiration and expiration because the immobilization in each case is in the position of normal movement.

An **inspiration bucket handle**[3] lesion is one in which any rib from the second to the tenth inclusive is so rotated on an axis drawn from the head of the rib to the side of the sternum that the rib is moved upward with its lower border turned outward and its outer surface upward.

In comparing the facets on the vertebral bodies and transverse processes for articulation with the heads and tubercles of the ribs, it may be seen that the facets for the third group of ribs are flat and will permit of a much wider range of motion. In inspiration, when the axis is antero-posterior, the two extremities

1. See Gray, ibid., p. 285, foot of the page.

2. As for example by leaning over a chair arm which holds a rib from participation in normal thoracic movement.

3. These lesions were named rotation rib lesions in the report of the nomenclature committee. The author prefers to retain the older name for the present. The definitions here given of these lesions are those adopted by the A. O. A. from its committee's report.

are fixed and the rib rotates upward at its middle, gliding upward on the transverse process, which sometimes presents a problem in correction for if the rib becomes securely lodged there, it is necessary to disengage it from that barrier first. This may be done as in other lesions of the second and third groups by making use of the elasticity of the rib compressing it at its angle and at its anterior extremity, when with a slight impetus[1] to guide it in the right direction it may be held until the adjustive movement is given.

The diagnosis of an inspiration bucket handle rib lesion may be determined as follows:

1. Restricted motion.
2. Widening of the interspace between the lesioned rib and the one below in the midaxillary line; interspaces at the vertebral and sternal ends not deviated from the normal.
3. Lower border of the rib in lesion turned outward and the outer surface turned upward.

CORRECTIVE MOVEMENTS

The principle of correction for an inspiration bucket handle lesion is downward rotation in the midaxillary line.

General Rules.—Disengagement of the upper edge of the rib from the under border of the rib beneath may be necessary preceding correction. It may be accomplished by sidebending or rotation to the opposite side with pressure applied[2] to the lesioned rib to separate it at the moment of upward movement of the rib above.

XII. Side-Pulling Movement.—The patient, B, is assumed to have an inspiration bucket handle lesion of the right ninth rib. He is asked to sit on a stool or a low table while O stands to his left and reaches around B with both arms, applying the right thumb as near to the vertebral extremity as possible, while with the left thumb pressure is put toward the anterior end of the rib, the middle finger of each hand lying above the upper border of the shaft as far out on the rib as possible. O springs the rib enough to know that his leverages are right and then pulls B sidewise toward him which spreads the vertebræ and ribs upon the left and approximates them somewhat upon the right. B is asked to take

1. This is called springing the rib.
2. That is, by springing the rib.

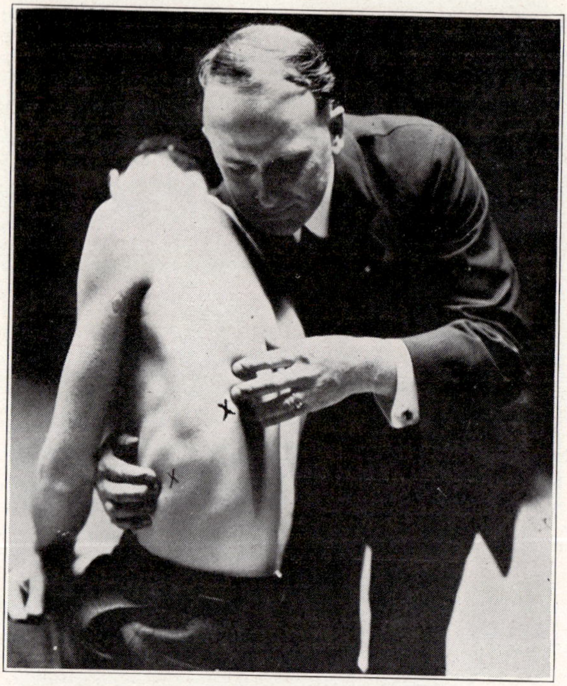

FIG. 69—Illustrating a corrective movement for an expiration bucket handle lesion of the left ninth rib, the interspace below the ninth represented by crosses.

a breath during the beginning of the sidewise movement and at its conclusion to exhale; toward the close of the expiration the adjustment is made.

An **expiration bucket handle** lesion is one in which any rib from the second to the tenth inclusive is so rotated on an axis from the head of the rib to the side of the sternum that the rib is moved downward with its upper border turned outward and its outer surface downward.[1]

CORRECTIVE MOVEMENTS

THE PRINCIPLE OF CORRECTION FOR AN EXPIRATION BUCKET HANDLE LESION IS UPWARD ROTATION ON THE ANTERO-POSTERIOR AXIS OF MOTION.

1. Definition of the committee on terminology before mentioned but with the name of rotated expiration lesion instead.

GENERAL RULES.—DISENGAGEMENT OF THE LOWER BORDER OF THE RIB FROM THE UPPER BORDER OF THE RIB BELOW MAY BE HAD BY SPRINGING THE RIB AND BY ROTATING THE PATIENT STRONGLY TO THE SIDE OPPOSITE THE LESION.

XIII. SIDE SPREADING MOVEMENT.—The patient, B, is assumed to have an expiration bucket handle lesion of the ninth left rib. B is asked to sit upon a stool or on the end of a low table, O standing beside him to the right. O takes hold of the rib as in the last corrective movement, and after springing it guides it upward at the centre while pushing B sidewise away from O thus lengthening the lateral wall[1] of the thorax on the side of the lesion and giving an added impulse to the intercostal muscle above the lesioned rib to contract.

LESIONS OF THE FOURTH GROUP OF RIBS

The eleventh and twelfth ribs differ from the others in that they are not as much curved, do not articulate by more than one

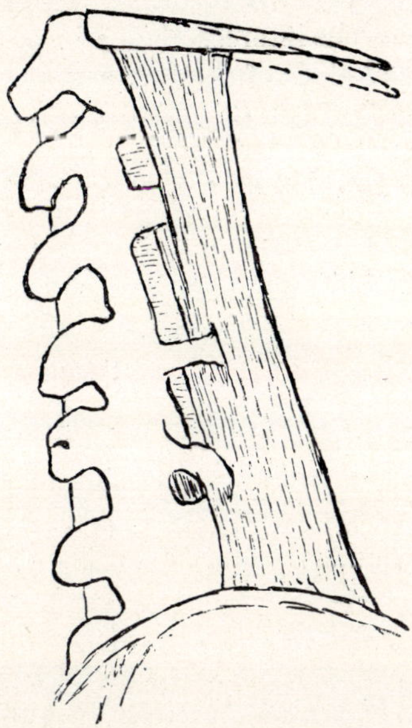

FIG. 70—Schematic drawing to illustrate the quadratus lumborum muscle and its action in connection with lesions of the twelfth rib. The dotted lines indicate the position of the rib when drawn down by this muscle.

1. Producing a convexity is not sufficient, for it may be seen that when B is sidebent to the right, a great deal of the side stretching comes in the lumbar area, affecting the eleventh and twelfth ribs and not those above especially.

joint with their respective vertebræ, have no tubercles, and no cartilaginous connection with other ribs, the cartilages of these terminating in the walls of the abdomen.

Lesions are caused by contraction of the quadratus lumborum upon the twelfth rib, by the pull of the lateral abdominal muscles, by traumatism, and, rarely, by forced respiratory movements.

The lesions[1] are upward or downward rotations. Normally the inner surface of the twelfth rib faces slightly upward. When an upward lesion occurs the twelfth rib is raised at its anterior extremity until often it has passed beneath the border of the eleventh, especially when the twelfth rib is unusually short. In downward displacements, the rib rotates slightly so that its inner surface faces inward and slightly downward and the anterior extremity of the rib is much depressed. The last intercostal muscle in such a case is thinned and atrophied.

The eleventh is subject to lesions in company with the twelfth, due to the tenacity of the intercostal muscle between them. There may be found these lesions of the last group of ribs:

1. Eleventh and twelfth ribs depressed, a lesion in which these ribs have been immobilized in a position of traumatic strain downward, with a slight rotation on a longitudinal axis in the same direction.
2. Eleventh and twelfth ribs raised, a lesion in which these ribs have been immobilized in a position of forced inspiration with some rotation on a longitudinal axis upward.
3. Twelfth rib depressed.
4. Twelfth rib raised.

The diagnosis of the depressed lesion of the twelfth rib may be established by the presence of the following signs:

1. Separation of the twelfth rib from the eleventh throughout its entire length but more especially at the costal extremity.
2. Restricted motion.

When the lesion is of the eleventh and twelfth, both depressed, the diagnosis is practically the same, restricted motion being the sign of lesion and separation between the upper border of the eleventh and the lower border of the tenth the evidence of a depressed lesion of these ribs.

1. The experiment described by C. P. McConnell (A. O. A. Jour., June, 1911, pg. 476, notes the effect of such lesions.

CORRECTIVE MOVEMENTS

The principle of correction for a depressed twelfth rib lesion is upward raising and inward rotation of the rib.

General Rule. — The quadratus lumborum muscle must be relaxed since its contraction is one of the factors maintaining lesion.

XIV. Quadratus Lumborum Movement.—The patient, B, is assumed to have a depressed lesion of the right twelfth rib. He is asked to lie supine on the table and flex his knees resting the feet on the table. O stands beside the table on B's left. He reaches around B's knees and takes hold of his legs so that he can swing them about, making a concavity on the left side, a convexity on the right, stretching the quadratus muscle, while he holds with his right hand the lesioned twelfth rib as a fixed insertion against which to stretch the muscle. Several leg-sidebendings may be necessary for this purpose.

O then passes his right hand under B's back until the middle finger presses against the rib at its vertebral extremity pushing it out into the abdominal wall. With his left hand O grasps the costal end and lower border of the rib and pulls it up to its accustomed place below the eleventh. Then holding the rib throughout

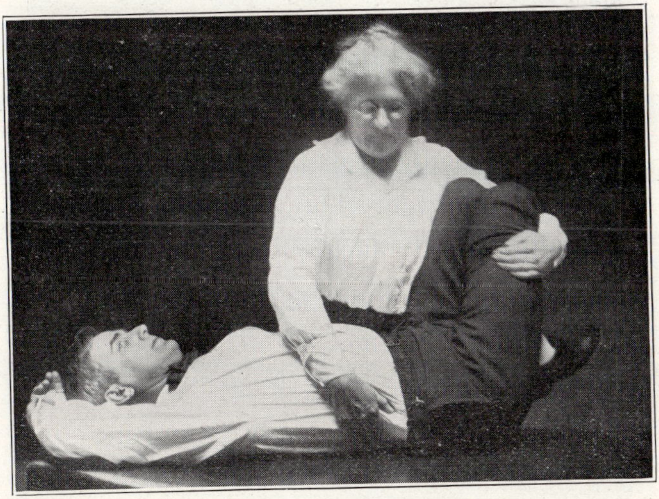

Fig. 71—Illustrating the method of stretching the quadratus lumborum muscle when lesion of the twelfth rib is present.

its length, O leans his right shoulder against B's chest to limit the upper excursion of the thorax while B takes a deep breath. The rib should be held thus for several moments while B repeats the deep inhalations.

XV. BIAS ROTATION MOVEMENT.—Let B lie upon the left side, while O stands behind him holding the twelfth rib upward in place, or holding the eleventh and twelfth when both are depressed, while his right elbow in front of B's right innominate and his left elbow behind B's shoulder, he is able to control a bias stretching of the quadratus lumborum and the lateral abdominal muscles. B is asked to assist by carrying his leg back and by rotating his right shoulder forward at the same time he takes a deep breath. O may reenforce his left hand with his right if he prefers.

XVI. SHOULDER-RAISING MOVEMENT.—Let the patient, B, who is assumed to have a depressed lesion of the right eleventh and

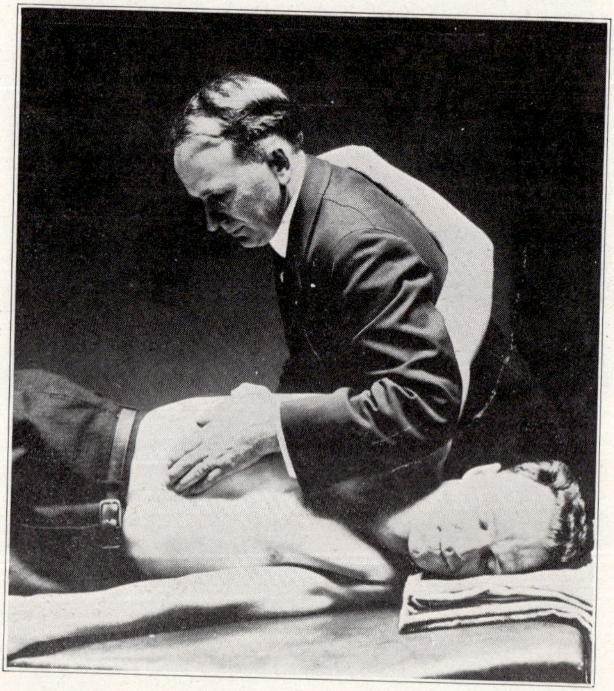

FIG. 72—Illustrating a method of raising all the ribs when liver treatment is indicated; or a manner of placing the patient for the adjustment of an expiration bucket handle lesion, or for lifting depressed eleventh and twelfth ribs.

twelfth ribs, lie upon his left side. O stands behind him and taking hold of B's right arm steps between it and his chest wall. He asks B to grasp his right shoulder so that O may by a backward bending lift all the ribs upon B's right chest wall through the pull of the muscles attached to the shoulder girdle. O faces B's feet and with his fingers under the under borders of the eleventh and twelfth ribs pulls them up while at the same time by some backward bending he raises all the ribs of the right wall of the thorax.

CORRECTIVE MOVEMENTS

The principle of correction for an elevated twelfth rib is separation from the eleventh with outward rotation.

General Rules.—Contraction of the intercostal muscles between the eleventh and twelfth ribs and atony of the quadratus lumborum muscle must be overcome.

XVII. Adhesion-Breaking Movement.—The patient, B, is assumed to have an upward lesion of the right twelfth rib, with the costal extremity of that rib held under the lower border of the eleventh. With the patient in the position of the quadratus lumborum movement, O reaches under B's back and pushes upward against the vertebral extremity of the twelfth rib, which is usually sufficient to carry its costal extremity out from under the border of the eleventh. O then grasps the end of it to hold the separation gained until O may place the tip of his middle finger between the eleventh and twelfth ribs at the vertebral end. O then places the left middle finger behind the right one pushing the right one slightly ahead. O then withdraws the right hand and places the middle finger behind the finger of the left hand and pushes that finger by slow steady movements forward in the effort to forcibly wedge the ribs apart and stretch the contracted intercostal muscle and break any connective tissue adhesions that may have formed.

Upward lesions of the eleventh and twelfth together may be treated in much the same way for the two ribs have seemed to move as one upward.

After the intercostal contractions have been overcome, O may place his right hand firmly against the lower border of the tenth rib, when the eleventh and twelfth are in lesion, or against the lower border of the eleventh when the twelfth only is in upward lesion, and using the first part of the quadratus lumborum movement, O may pull the ribs below the fixed point downward and assist in correcting the lesion.

The shoulder-raising movement may be used in the same way by placing the hand underneath the lowest rib not in lesion and by the upward pulling of the lateral thoracic wall stretch the intercostal muscle in contraction. O may place his thumb close to the vertebral border of the rib between it and the rib above and gradually wedge it forward using shoulder-raising in conjunction.

AFTER-TREATMENT

The first requirement for the maintenance of rib correction is proper respiratory action. Breathing correctly done helps to establish a normal equilibrium and also to maintain the flexibility of the segments of the thoracic area of the spine. Especially should the physician inquire into the habitual sitting position of the patient for those of sedentery life are notoriously poor breathers. Examination of the upper air passages should be made to discover any obstructions that might impede respiration.

The importance of these lesions should need no demonstration to those who remember that the thoracic ganglia lie on the anterior surfaces of the heads of the ribs. The researches of Dr. Louisa Burns of "The A. T. Still Research Institute" of Chicago have confirmed clinical evidence that the blood content is changed after the correction of rib lesions.

THE STRAIGHT SPINE AND THE FLAT CHEST

The patient who suffers from having a straight spine and a flat chest upon physical examination presents the following clinical signs: decreased pelvic inclination, straight lumbar area, flat dorsal region,[1] straight cervical area; winged scapulæ; decreased antero-posterior diameter of the thorax and increased transverse diameter of the same; arms seemingly longer than the normal; in men, prominence of the crico-thyroid cartilages. The symptoms of which they complain are lowered resistance with a tendency to catching cold, catarrhal predisposition, bronchitis, and influenza; they are easily affected by the stimuli of environment, barometric changes, season, altitude; neurasthenia with its concomitant symptoms of irritability, dyspepsia, vaso-motor dis-

1. This has been spoken of as the anterior dorsal in our earlier literature.

turbances. It seems impossible for them to remain well long at a time, respiration is insufficient, they suffer from malnutrition, and even though ambitious want the necessary energy to accomplish more than the average quota of achievement. They are subject to nervous disturbances in consequence of the rigidity which is often present in pelvic and spinal articulations, resulting in constant jarring[1] of the highly sensitive nervous tissues.

The flat chest[2] is characterized by an increase in obliquity of the ribs, of the fourth to the seventh in particular, with narrowed interspaces, sternal and vertebral ends closer together with increased curving[3] laterally. The subcostal angle is less than a right angle. It is in large measure due to the change in the shape of the ribs that the dorsal spine becomes straight. A flat dorsal area upon close examination of the spine of the cadaver, shows more or less extension of each of the thoracic vertebral joints, with subsequent narrowing of intervertebral foraminæ and impaired circulation to the spinal centres, which, in the area of vasomotor control, is full of suggestion as to consequences.

The causes of this condition are many: first may be mentioned the influence of heredity predisposing to weakness and insufficient muscular strength to avoid the pitfalls of faulty attitudes and habits; secondly, infectious conditions which through sequent weakness predispose to the same condition, as pneumonia, the exanthemata in severe form, tuberculosis and pleurisy in adults, and any irritative process which may immobilize the chest wall as herpes zoster, fractured ribs, pleural adhesions; it is directly caused by disturbances in equilibrium, as accompanying extension lesions of the sacrum[4], injuries to the cervical or upper dorsal regions, or resultant upon extreme weakness in children who are sent to school and told to stand erect with shoulders back, a pernicious order aggravating the real condition instead of ameliorating it. Obstructive hindrances to breathing, such as adenoids, nasal polypi, enlarged turbinates, predispose to lessened

1. See page 135, paragraph 1.
2. The flat chest has been designated in the older medical literature as the paralytic, phthisinoid, and phthisical chest.
3. The shape of the ribs actually changes, the curve is more pronounced and the obliquity greater.
4. See pg. 135, paragraph 2.

respiration, secondarily poor habits of breathing and impaired capacity of the lungs, after which naturally follows a diminution in the diameters of the chest.

The diagnosis rests upon the presence of the signs and symptoms above described.

CORRECTIVE MOVEMENTS

THE PRINCIPLES OF CORRECTION FOR A STRAIGHT SPINE AND A FLAT CHEST ARE RESTORATION OF EACH SPINAL AREA TO ITS NORMAL PHYSIOLOGICAL CURVE; OF EACH VERTEBRAL, RIB, AND SACRO-ILIAC ARTICULATION TO ITS NORMAL MOTION; OF EACH RIB TO ITS NORMAL FORM AND POSITION.

GENERAL RULES.—THE AREAS OF THE SPINE SHALL BE CONSIDERED AS SEPARATE GROUP LESIONS WITH TREATMENT DIRECTED IN ACCORD WITH THAT IDEA. EACH DORSAL SEGMENT SHALL BE TREATED IN TURN. THE SACRUM SHALL BE REGARDED AS AN EXTENSION SACRAL LESION AND SHALL BE ADJUSTED BY FLEXION OF THE SACRUM OR EXTENSION OF BOTH INNOMINATES. THE BEND SHALL BE REDUCED IN EACH RIB BY A COMBINATION OF COMPRESSION AND STIMULATION OF NORMAL EXPANSION; BY THE LATTER MEANS THE RIB WILL BE RAISED TO ITS NORMAL POSITION, FOR A RIB PREVENTED FROM EXPANDING IN ONE DIRECTION WILL EXPAND IN ANOTHER.

The patient must be examined thoroughly for organic conditions which may be predisposing to the continuation of the condition. Adenoid tissue must be removed when it exists in the upper air passages. Lack of proper hygienic surroundings and occupation must be remedied. If the patient is young and frail the treatment must be very carefully administered for with these patients at any age the resistance is so much lowered that cure is a slow process. They should be told frankly that there is no easy road to recovery and that it will require patience on the part both of physician and patient.

Examination should be made for spinal and rib lesions for any additional exciting cause must be removed before the specific treatment can avail much. Between treatments the patient should assume as often as possible the proper standing position with the weight on the balls of the feet, the lumbar area in forward extension. All patients under thirty years of age, without organic conditions, should be cured. Patients over thirty may be helped.

XVIII. EXPANSION TRANSVERSE COMPRESSION MOVEMENT.—Let the patient, B, lie upon the table in the position described in experimental palpation, F, page 98. Let O take the same relative position to B and, placing his right arm under B's lateral thoracic wall, rest the right palm over the ribs that lie just below the scapula in the posterior axillary line, reenforcing the pressure with the left hand over the right. O then places his chest against the right anterior axillary line in a direct diagonal line from the hands. B then turns his chest forward toward the ventral position and is instructed to take a full breath and hold it as long as possible. O begins at the middle of B's inhalation to exert pressure between his hands and the chest, maintaining the pressure while B holds his breath and then relaxing it rapidly as B exhales. While B is holding his breath and O is maintaining the

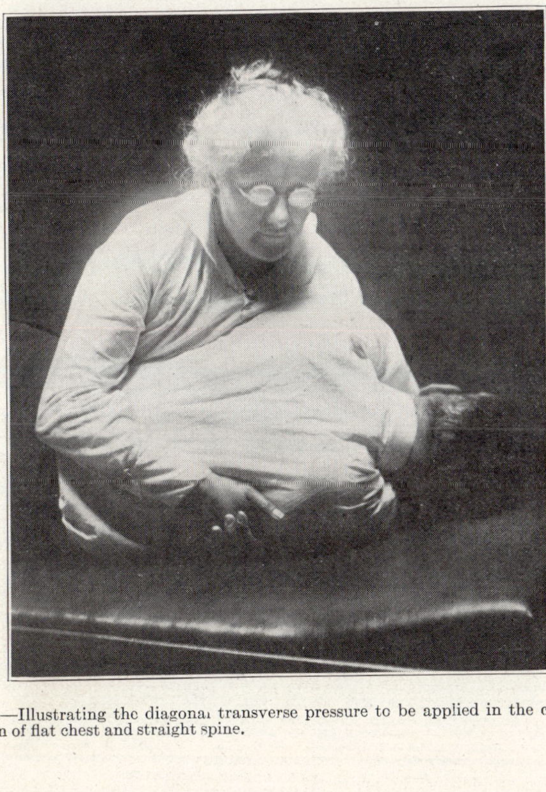

FIG. 73—Illustrating the diagonal transverse pressure to be applied in the correction of the condition of flat chest and straight spine.

pressure, O adds a slight rotation of B's torso backward, but not passing the direct lateral position, at which point pressure and respiratory expansion are greatest. This movement should be repeated nine times upon each side. The spine should be bared that O may observe the effect upon the thoracic vertebræ.

The amount of pressure exerted should be increased as the patient continues treatment, beginning with only a few foot-pounds of pressure at first and then as the condition improves making use of more constraint in the diagonal diameter. The caution to be observed is that pressure shall not be applied before B has produced quite a little thoracic expansion and that the compression shall not be unbearable at any time in the treatment of the case. The movements will need to be repeated at different levels if the entire thorax is involved.

The same movement may be given with the patient sitting on a stool leaning against the wall or in the case of a child against the table. O in either case kneels to bring his chest at a proper level for compression.

The same movement may be used for the correction of thoracic functional curvature by having the patient lie upon the side of the convexity and giving the movement to expand the chest in the opposite diagonal diameter.

A similar operation is made for the assistance of a heart which is dilated and needs more room. It may be described, thus:

XIX. CAPACITY INCREASING MOVEMENT.—Let B, the patient, who is assumed to have a heart in the state of dilatation or uncompensated hypertrophy to whom some relief may be given by more room on the left side of the thorax, lie supine upon the table. O stands to his right and places his left hand underneath B's back until the palmar surface of the hand rests against the posterior axillary line in the area of the left fifth to eighth ribs. O reenforces the right hand with the left which is passed across the abdomen. O places his chest against the anterior axillary line on the right and makes diagonal transverse compression while B holds a full breath, relaxing the pressure as B expires. It may be necessary to give B resting periods between the corrective movements and his position may be varied to suit the circumstances. The principle of correction remains the same, the production of functional curvature convex to the right so that diagonally across the thorax there will be bulging anteriorly.

CHAPTER IX

OCCIPITO-ATLANTAL LESIONS

The articulations between the occiput[1] and atlas and between the atlas and axis are classed as diarthroses, freely movable joints. The occipito-atlantal joints are called condylarthroses because the articulating surfaces are the condyles of the occiput and the superior facets of the atlas. There are three arthrodial joints between the atlas and axis, two being formed by articular facets, the third, a trochoid or pivot-joint, formed by the dens articulating with the anterior arch of the atlas in front and with the transverse ligament behind.

Briefly reviewed, the condyles of the occiput are oval in form, convexo-convex so that facing downward they also face forward, backward, and outward. They do not lie parallel to each other save in those people of different races who have borne weights upon their heads. Almost always the condyles converge toward each other anteriorly and diverge from each other posteriorly.

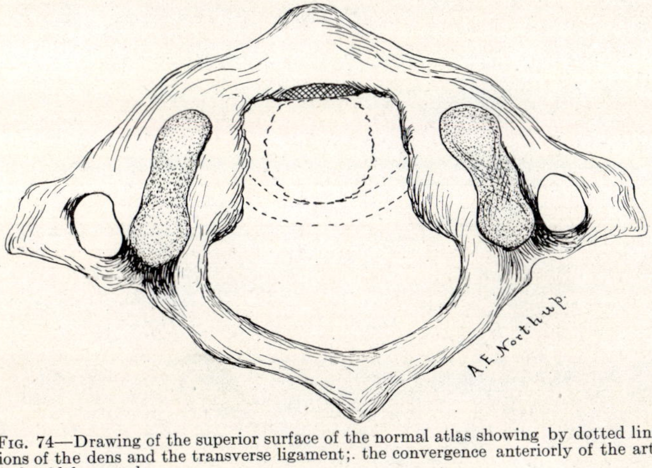

FIG. 74—Drawing of the superior surface of the normal atlas showing by dotted lines the positions of the dens and the transverse ligament;. the convergence anteriorly of the articular facets should be noted.

1. In osteopathic literature the word occiput is used interchangeably with occipital bone.

The superior articular facets of the atlas correspond in shape and relation to the condyles of the occipital bone. They are concavo-concave and the posterior margins are on a slightly lower level than the anterior ones. They face upward, medially, and slightly forward and backward.

The movements of the atlas upon the axis have been well understood by anatomists for years but of the movements of the occiput upon the atlas little is known beyond flexion and extension. Lateral bending has been recognized lately but rotation is practically unknown.[1]

FLEXION OF THE OCCIPUT

Flexion is accomplished in the occipito-atlantal articulation by a moving of the condyle backward, downward, and inward upon the corresponding facet of the atlas, explained in detail, thus: when the top of the head moves forward both condyles glide backward and since they converge anteriorly their anterior extremities in moving backward must encroach upon the lateral masses of the atlas internal to the facets, and also, because the facets slope downward, the condyles must glide downward. When they come to rest, the posterior one-third of each condylar surface projects beyond the posterior margin of each facet; the remaining part of each condyle rests upon the inner one-half of the posterior two-thirds of each facet. The axis of motion is a transverse one represented by a line which passes through the jugular processes of the occipital bone, in the average individual.

---

1. It is a strange fact but nevertheless true that syndesmology has been given less of exhaustive study than any of the other systems of the human body save where a joint has had surgical importance. Even in a text as standard as Cunningham's Anatomy, seven pages will be given to a presentation of the knee-joint while one and one-half pages will suffice to cover the articulations of the occiput, the most important of the body. Since the science of osteopathy has brought to the attention of more than one thinking orthopedist the function of the sacro-iliac joint, it is safe to predict that in less than a decade orthopedists will have observed more closely occipital and cervical lesions and in consequence there may be found comprehensive descriptions of all the articulations in every text-book that treats of human syndesmology.

Bibliography: Cunningham, ibid., p. 309-311.
Deaver, ibid., Vol. I., p. 417-424.
Gray, ibid., p. 273-278.
Morris, ibid., p. 218-224.
Jour. of the A. O. A., Dec., 1908, p. 168; Jan. 1909, p. 210; April, 1909, p. 344.

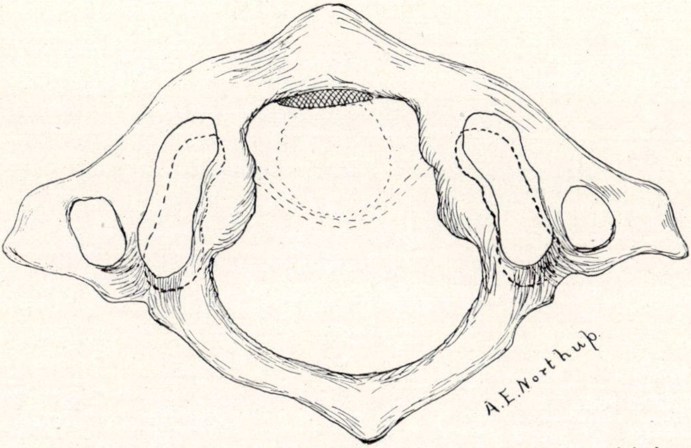

FIG. 75—Drawing to represent by heavy dotted lines the position of the occipital condyles in slight flexion of the occiput.

The amount of movement in extreme occipito-atlantal flexion has been variously estimated and scarcely two observers are agreed upon the amount of gliding that takes place. It seems reasonable to conclude, after close study of the two bones entering into the articulation and with due consideration to the number of limiting ligaments and muscles about the joint, that a gliding of more than one-quarter of an inch is unlikely if not impossible; the extent of the motion may be even less. In some cases an elongated dens would prevent greater flexion, in fact it is not uncommon for an articulation to be found between the apex of the dens on its forward edge and the anterior rim of the foramen magnum, shown by the presence of articular facets, small in size, upon these bones.

Immobilization of the articulations in flexion would result in the formation of a flexion lesion, called in osteopathic terminology a posterior occiput.[1] The causes of such a lesion would be inflammation from infectious diseases, toxins, or as a result of strain; contraction leading to contracture of the flexor muscles; atony of the extensor muscles following long continued faulty posture in

1. A large number of osteopathists still use the term, anterior atlas, to designate this lesion. Since the upper of the bones entering into a vertebral joint is the movable one, the name should be that of the upper bone, and this applies to the occipito-atlantal articulations quite as much if not more than to any other spinal joint.

consequence of refractive errors, thoracic kyphosis with accentuation of the cervical curve, etc.

EXPERIMENTAL PALPATION, O.—The presence or absence of motion in the occipito-atlantal articulation may be determined by palpation only. Let the subject, B, who has normal articulations between the occiput and the atlas, sit upon a stool, with O standing behind him. For convenience, three points may be chosen from which to estimate whether or not movement is present in the articulation under consideration. These points are the posterior border of the ramus of the mandible at a point adjacent to the transverse process of the atlas which is the second point in the process of comparison; the third point is the tip of the mastoid process of the temporal bone. Let O place the radial side of the index finger against the transverse process of the atlas letting the nail rest against the ramus anterior and the surface of the finger also rest against the mastoid process at the tip. If the articulation is normal, O will find that there is some separation between the anterior border of the transverse process and the ramus while the tip of the mastoid lies just above or slightly in front of the posterior border of the transverse process. For comparison of the relation of the tip of the mastoid to the posterior border of the transverse process of the atlas, separately, O may place the palmar surface of the thumb against these and palpate their contiguous surfaces.

Now let O place both index fingers in position for palpating to determine movement, and ask B to flex the head forward whereupon O may observe that the distance between the ramus of the mandible and the anterior border of the transverse process has become narrowed and that the tip of the mastoid has moved behind the posterior border of the transverse process. B is asked to raise his head, whereupon the three points resume their normal relations.

Since a flexion lesion signifies immobilization in a position of flexion, two signs of such an occipital lesion would be approximation of the ramus and transverse process and separation of the latter and the tip of the mastoid, the mastoid being posterior.

EXPERIMENTAL PALPATION, P.—Let B, the patient, be one who is assumed to have a posterior occipital lesion. O standing behind B with fingers applied to his occipital area as in the first part of the above experiment, notes that the ramus is approximated to the transverse process so that the finger tip may not be placed between them. O asks B to extend his head backward, and notes no resulting change in the relation of the processes.

He is asked to flex his head forward but with no movement in the articulation apparent. From the absence of motion O may conclude that lesion is present.

If, however, when B bends his head backward, a separation appears between the anterior border of the transverse process and the ramus an anomalous condition may be present.

The atlas is often found to have transverse processes that do not conform to the general rules of proportion for the parts of that bone. Its transverse processes may be exceedingly small so that they cannot be palpated laterally; they may be very large so that they are level upon their outer surfaces with the mastoids and the lateral surfaces of the rami; they may be irregular, having one large and one small transverse process, or one large and the other normal, or one small and the other normal, or with irregular borders, the anterior border upon one side being large, upon the opposite side small. The sign of lesion,[1] it must not be forgotten, is restricted mobility, hence the only test of an anomalous bone as a part of an articulation is motion.

A **bilaterally posterior occipital** lesion is one in which the occipito-atlantal articulations are immobilized in the position of flexion.

Since contraction of the flexors produces normal flexion, when lesion is present the flexors are contracted, the extensors stretched. Subsequent changes in these muscles will be shown in thickening and shortening of the flexors and atrophy and thinning of the extensors. The ligaments anterior to the articulations of the occiput and atlas and the occiput and axis will be shortened and thickened, the posterior ligaments stretched.

A head immobilized in flexion with one vertebra will not remain in that position long, but will by the accentuation of the cervical curve or by the production of two or more cervical lesions restore erectness to itself. Lesions, whether by group or singly, thus produced, are at first compensatory or counterbalancing

1. There may be a lesion of a vertebra having anomalous processes which would of course be confusing but in such a case the operative measures would be in the line of securing motion through putting the articulation through a full range of movement followed by corrective movements for the suspected lesion, which, if it fails of correction after a reasonable number of trials, would indicate that re-examination should be made and with the possibility of an anomaly present, it may be decided to change the operative technique.

lesions, but due to the weight of the head and the strain of holding it upright, contraction of muscles in unbalance causes the lesions to be in effect the same as primary ones.

These lesions are fairly common, the most common of the occipital group of lesions. The almost constant symptom of which these patients complain is an uneasiness at the back of the neck close to the occiput due unquestionably to the extra strain upon the extensor muscles that any labor which is performed with the head in flexion would subject them to. In patients who have acute lesions or are frail or sick, tenderness about the articulations is often found.

CORRECTIVE MOVEMENTS

THE PRINCIPLE OF CORRECTION FOR A FLEXION LESION OF THE OCCIPITO-ATLANTAL ARTICULATION IS EXTENSION.

GENERAL RULES.—SINCE EACH OCCIPITAL CONDYLE HAS MOVED INWARD AND DOWNWARD AS WELL AS BACKWARD, IT MUST BE MOVED IN CORRECTION OUTWARD, FORWARD, AND UPWARD; THEREFORE THE OPERATIVE PROCEDURE FOR THE ADJUSTMENT OF A POSTERIOR OCCIPUT MUST BE GIVEN TO ONE ARTICULATION AT A TIME.

Preliminary treatment is almost a necessity in these cases for in the presence of a number of small contractured muscles it is difficult to secure an adjustment early in the treatment of the articulation. By putting the cervical region through its normal movements, with especial effort to separate the origin and insertion of all muscles of length attached to the occiput, atlas, or axis, preparation is made for localizing the operative work at the occipito-atlantal articulation. An attempt should then be made to put the joint through its normal range of movement but by gentle means, after which the corrective work should be given.

I. OUTWARD EXTENSION MOVEMENT.—Let B, the patient, lie supine upon the table, with his head projecting beyond the end of the table. O stands at his head and with a pillow between his abdomen and the top of B's head places pressure against the top of his head to hold it in the plane with his body. O places his hands overlapped under B's head with the thumbs resting against the determining points for observation[1], or at least between the

1. For the purpose of detecting when movement begins; at that time is the operative procedure effective.

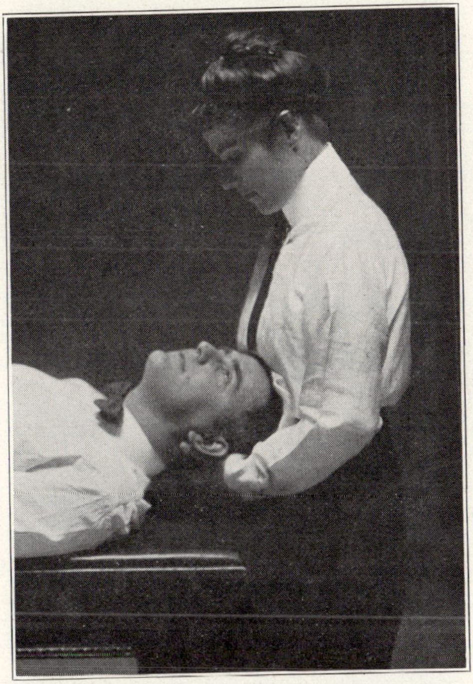

FIG. 76—Illustrating the position of patient and physician at the beginning of the head-extension movement for correction of the flexion lesion of the occiput.

transverse process and the ramus, with very light pressure, not sufficient to cause the patient the least annoyance and never with the idea of fixing the atlas or of moving it.

O lifts B's head in slight extension by raising the chin just a little and depressing the occiput. He then carries B's chin straight to the right without any rotation of his face. By these two movements he has directed the right condyle forward and outward. By an increase of pressure upon the top of B's head, O lifts it in extension which should adjust the condyle to the facet if there be no extensive shortening of the anterior ligaments or calcareous deposit[1] about the articulation. Holding the extension, O carries B's chin back to the median line and, bending his own knees slightly, he lowers B's head as a whole. The movement is then repeated with change of direction to the left. Throughout the movement

1. Crepitus is the sign of such deposit about the articulation. The patient often complains of grating sounds heard when the head is moved. The physician notes them in corrective movements given the patient.

there is no rotation of the head nor is there any change of the top of the head from the median line of the body.

Several repetitions should be made to each side. The adjustment is not easily made nor is it possible to hold the correction obtained at any treatment unless with the cooperation of the patient who avoids flexion of the head as much as possible between treatments or counterbalances it by extension against resistance to give strength to the extensor muscles. When the joints have attained a normal range of movement, adjustment may be said to be complete.

The counterpart of this movement may be given with the patient seated upon a stool. There are variations in the positions of the hands which may suggest themselves to the physician as more suitable to his habit.

EXTENSION OF THE OCCIPUT

Extension is accomplished in the occipito-atlantal articulation by a moving of the condyle forward, upward, and outward upon the corresponding facet of the atlas, explained in detail, thus; when the top of the head moves backward both condyles glide forward and since they diverge posteriorly, their outer margins must overhang the lateral edges of the facets, so that they glide outward as well as forward. Since the anterior extremity of each facet is on a higher level than the posterior part, the condyle also moves upward. When the joints come to a position of rest in extension, the posterior two-thirds of each condyle by the inner half of its surface rests upon the outer half of the anterior two-thirds of each articular facet. They move upon the transverse axis of motion and the extent of the movement is no greater than it is in flexion, although provision has been made in the posterior condylar fossæ for the reception of the posterior margins of the articular facets in extension. The depth and size of these fossæ indicate that the movement is not large.

Immobilization of the articulation in extension would constitute the bilateral anterior occipital lesion. The causes of the production of this lesion are inflammation, after the manner of the invasion of any joint, contraction of the extensor muscles, atony of the flexors, weakness resulting in postural defects such as round shoulders making it a necessity for the subject to raise the head back in extension to look at objects upon the horizon. It is found in very young children before the development of the normal physiological curves is complete; it is often found in an old person counterbalancing dorsal kyphosis.

EXPERIMENTAL PALPATION, Q.—Let the subject, B, sit upon a stool, O standing behind him with his index fingers applied to B's neck as in experimental palpation, O. B is asked to carry his head back in extension, whereupon O should note that there is marked separation between the ramus and the anterior border of the transverse process; that the tip of the mastoid has moved forward until it overhangs the anterior border of the transverse process. Ask B to resume the erect position of his head and the distance will return to the normal between the ramus and the transverse process.

Palpating the posterior borders of the transverse processes in relation to the mastoid processes with the palmar surfaces of the thumbs, the difference is easily detected between the position in extension and the normal erect position.

EXPERIMENTAL PALPATION, R.—Let the patient, B, be assumed to have an extension lesion of the occiput. Ask him to sit as in the preceding experiment upon the stool, O standing behind him and palpating the ramus of the mandible and the transverse process to diagnose the condition of each occipito-atlantal articulation. O asks B to bend his head forward in flexion. There is no change in the relations of the ramus, mastoid, and transverse process, the ramus and transverse process being separated, the

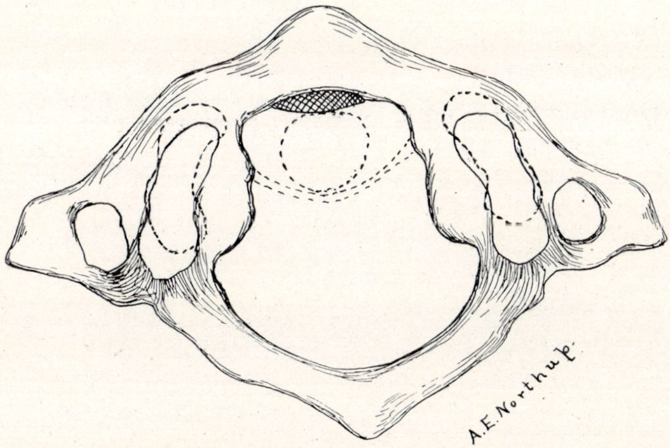

FIG. 77—Drawing to represent by heavy dotted lines the position of the occipital condyles in moderate extension of the occiput.

transverse and mastoid approximated. B is then asked o extend the head and again no change is detected, not even an increase in the signs of the lesion.

The diagnosis of the extension lesion is the presence of the distinctive signs upon each side:

1. Restricted motion.
2. Separation of the ramus of the mandible from the anterior border of the transverse process of the atlas.
3. Approximation of the tip of the mastoid and the anterior border of the transverse process.
4. Straightening of the cervical curve, an effort at counterbalance.

A bilateral anterior occiput may be defined as a subluxation, or immobilization, of the occipito-atlantal articulations in the position of extension.

The pathological changes about the joints are contracture of the extensor muscles, atony of the flexors, calcareous deposit,[1] shortening of the posterior ligaments, and stretching of the anterior and lateral occipito-atlantal and the apical dental ligaments. These lesions are very uncommon and set up no definite train of symptoms distinguishable from those found in other occipito-atlantal lesions.

CORRECTIVE MOVEMENTS

THE PRINCIPLE OF CORRECTION FOR AN OCCIPITO-ATLANTAL EXTENSION LESION IS FLEXION.

GENERAL RULES.—SINCE EACH OCCIPITAL CONDYLE HAS MOVED FORWARD, UPWARD AND OUTWARD UPON THE FACET, IT MUST BE MOVED DOWNWARD, BACKWARD, AND INWARD IN CORRECTION. THE OPERATIVE PROCEDURE FOR ADJUSTMENT OF THE ANTERIOR OCCIPUT MUST BE GIVEN TO ONE ARTICULATION AT A TIME.

Preliminary treatment is an essential part in the correction of any occipital lesion, and that which has been described for the treatment of a posterior occiput applies to an anterior, lateral, or rotated occiput as well.

1. See the author's article, "Osteological Proofs", in the Jour. of the A. O. A., July, 1914.

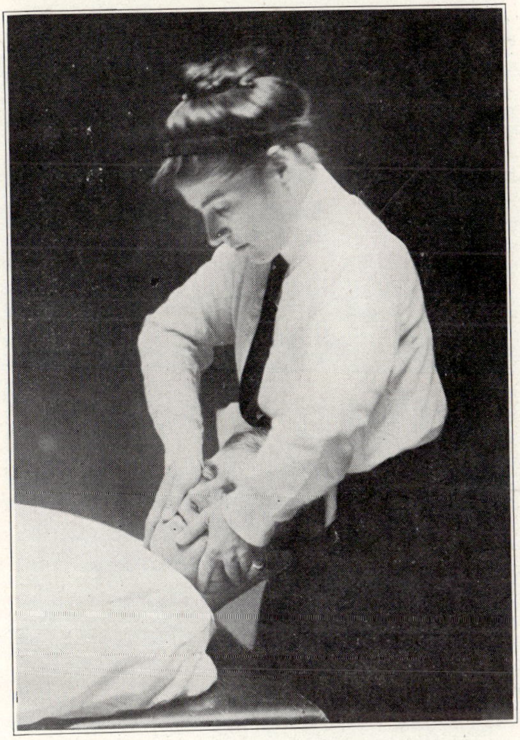

FIG. 78—Illustrating the position of patient and physician at the beginning of the head-flexion movement for the correction of the extension lesion of the occiput.

II. OUTWARD FLEXION MOVEMENT.—Let the patient, B, lie supine upon the table as in the outward flexion movement with O standing in the same relative position to B.

O places his abdomen against the pillow which he places between B's head and the pressure directed through O's body to the top of B's head. O rises slightly upon his toes until he has lifted B's occiput and depressed his chin slightly. He then places the heels of his hands upon B's malar bones with the fingers directed downward, the middle fingers palpating the posterior borders and adjacent surfaces of the mastoid processes, for the purpose of detecting when correction has begun in the articulations.

O carries B's chin to the left without moving the top of his head from the mesial plane, or turning his face. O then puts an additional pressure downward through the malar bones at the same time rising a little more upon his toes, adding to the amount of flexion already attempted in the joints by position. The pressure and position are held while the chin is returned to the median line, whereupon the pressure is relaxed through the hands, and the physician lessens the degree of rising upon his feet, until the position is the same with which the movement started. The movement is then repeated in the opposite direction.

Several repetitions should be made to each side. The palpating fingers will be able to determine when movement begins in the joints. Between treatments the patient may assist by exercising the atonic flexors by resistance exercises.

Following adjustment, the articulations should be put through their range of movements again and again until each is known to be normal. It is then that the lesion has been completely adjusted.

SIDEBENDING OF THE OCCIPUT

Lateral gliding of the occiput upon the atlas has been described in Morris's Anatomy, in several editions, as a "sinking of the lateral edge of one condyle a little within the lateral edge of the socket of the atlas" with the "opposite condyle projecting to a corresponding degree." The top of "the head is thus tilted to one side and it is even possible that the weight of the skull may be borne almost entirely on one joint."

In sidebending of the top of the head to the right, the right condyle glides downward and inward upon the right articular facet and the left condyle glides upward and outward upon its corresponding facet, but the extent of the movement is much less than takes place in flexion and extension, being perhaps not greater than one-eighth of an inch in extreme lateral flexion, its movement limited by the left alar and the left anterior oblique ligaments. Its axis of motion is an antero-posterior one.

When the occiput becomes immobilized in the position of right sidebending from any of the causes operative in producing subluxation, such as trauma, inflammation, faulty posture, refractive error, contracture and atony of muscles, the top of the head is bent away from the horizontal plane and the first effort on the part of the individual thus afflicted is to make erect the head, by producing a cervical curve, convex on the side on which the condyle has sunk, concave on the other side, or by the production of a secondary atlas lesion, or when the lateral occipital

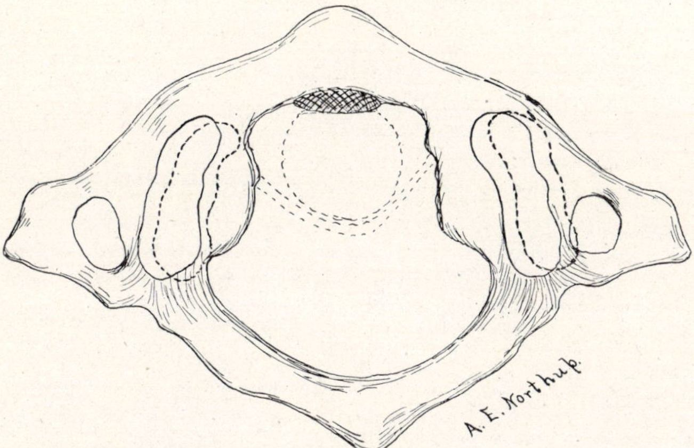

FIG. 79—Drawing to represent by heavy dotted lines the position of the occipital condyles in left sidebending of the occiput.

lesion is slight in extent by a cervical lesion, anterior to the same side.

The lesion is termed an occiput lateral to the left, named from the prominence of the mastoid process which in sidebending to the right is carried upward and outward upon the left.

EXPERIMENTAL PALPATION, S.—Let the subject, B, sit upon a stool behind which O stands, with his index fingers palpating the area of the transverse processes of the atlas and the mastoid processes of the temporals. He then asks B to sidebend his head to the right, whereupon O should detect that the tip of the right mastoid has moved slightly to the left and has approached vertically the transverse process so that it is not difficult for the palpating finger to note the difference between the lateral position and the normal. Upon the left, the tip of the mastoid projects laterally in a noticeable manner beyond the lateral edge of the transverse process and it is also separated vertically from it.

Immobilization of the occipito-atlantal articulation in the position of right sidebending would be the definition of a left lateral occiput and from the experimental palpation above, the diagnosis may be deduced:

1. Restricted motion.
2. Separation of the tip of the right mastoid from the transverse process below with lateral projection of the mastoid.
3. Approximation of the tip of the left mastoid and the transverse process with lack of prominence laterally of the mastoid.
4. The presence of counterbalancing lesions.

CORRECTIVE MOVEMENTS

THE PRINCIPLE OF CORRECTION FOR A LATERAL OCCIPITAL LESION IS SIDEBENDING TO THE SAME SIDE.

GENERAL RULES.—SINCE THE LESION IS PRODUCED IN SIDEBENDING TO ONE SIDE, CORRECTION MUST NECESSARILY BE MADE BY SIDEBENDING TO THE OPPOSITE SIDE AND SINCE EACH CERVICAL ARTICULATION ON THE SIDE OF THE CONCAVITY MAY MOVE BUT ONE-SIXTEENTH OF AN INCH, CORRECTION WILL BE EASILY LOCALIZED IN THE OCCIPTIO-ATLANTAL ARTICULATION BY EXTREME SIDEBENDING.

III. CONDYLE-SINKING MOVEMENT.—Let the patient, B, who is assumed to have a left lateral occiput lesion, lie supine upon the table, with his head projecting a few inches beyond the table

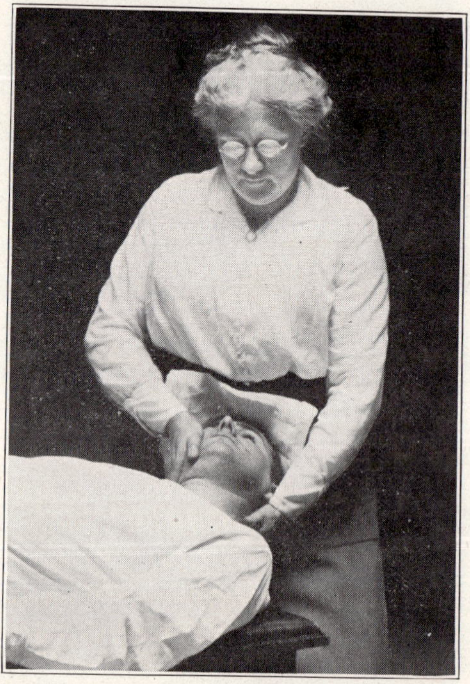

FIG. 80—Illustrating the position of patient and physician at the beginning of the condyle-sinking movement for the correction of the right lateral occipital lesion.

and resting against O's abdomen, a pillow interposed between. O places his left hand on B's cheek for the purpose of moving the head as a whole to the right. O's right hand is placed under the right side of the head so that it may be said to grasp the right mastoid process in the operative movement and to pull it upward as in a sidebending movement to the left.

O bends B's head to the left not turning the face in rotation. After some preliminary sidebending to each side with pressure maintained throughout upon the top of the head, O carries the head in extreme sidebending and then alternately adds a considerable amount of pressure in a straight line toward the right shoulder and relaxes it until when O is satisfied that B has relaxed perfectly. Then with increased pressure against the left cheek, increased pulling upward upon the right side of the head, O gives a sudden forcible pressure against the top of the head which is usually effective in adjusting the occiput to the atlas. The popping sound is ordinarily heard during this correction. O holds the head securely in his hands and then carries it to the mesial plane of the body and keeping it horizontal with pressure against the top of the head O alternately gives traction and adds pressure in a straight line downward toward B's feet, after which B is commanded to sidebend the head to the left against resistance several times in the effort to secure enough contraction in the atonic lateral muscles to hold the correction gained.

Practically the same movement may be given with the patient sitting on a stool, O standing back of B and slightly to his right. O places his left forearm over B's head, his hand under B's chin. B's right hand rests against the right side of the neck to help to localize the movement in the occipito-atlantal articulation. The operative movement is conducted as above.

The lateral occiput is third in frequency among occipital lesions, being more common than the anterior occiput but less frequent than the rotated occiput. It is somewhat easily adjusted.

The after-treatment accorded this lesion is practically the same as that indicated for any other occipital lesion. If there is a cause that can be removed aside from that local to the joint, removal is the necessary procedure.

ROTATION OF THE OCCIPUT

Due to the obliquity of the planes of the superior articular facets of the atlas, rotation of the occiput does not take place upon a horizontal plane. There are elements of flexion, extension, and

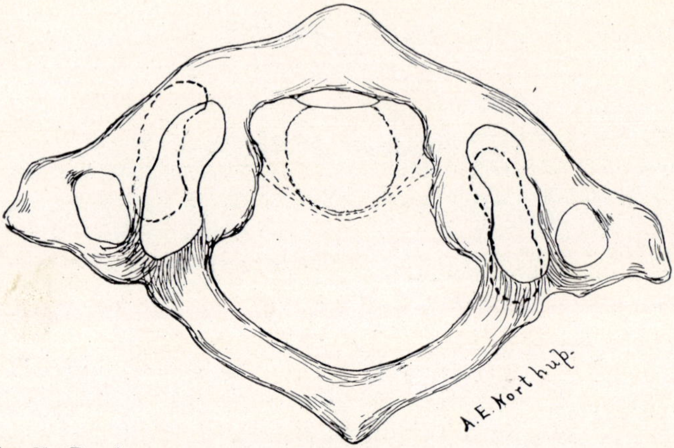

FIG. 81—Drawing to represent by heavy dotted lines the positions of the occipital condyles in rotation to the right of the occipito-atlantal joint.

sidebending in the movement. When the occiput is rotated to the right, the right condyle moves not only backward but also downward and inward; the left condyle moves not only forward but outward and upward. A horizontal place projected from the crown of the head would, by rotation of the occiput to the right, be tilted downward and backward on the same side.

EXPERIMENTAL PALPATION, T.—Let the subject, B, sit upon a stool behind which O stands with his hands placed for palpation as in the preceding experiments of this chapter. B is asked to turn his face to the right. O should note that the distance between the ramus of the mandible and the anterior border of the transverse process in narrowed upon the right, while upon the left it is noticeably widened. Upon the right the vertical distance between the tip of the mastoid and the lateral edge of the transverse process is slightly less than when the head is held erect, while upon the left the distance between the same two points is somewhat greater. Let B return his face to the front and then rotate his head to the left, whereupon the reverse of the preceding observations may be made.

Upon the presence of the above distinguishing signs may diagnosis of a rotated occiput be made when in addition there is restriction of motion and the presence of counterbalancing lesions in the atlo-axoid or other cervical articulations.

A rotation lesion of the occipito-atlantal articulations may be defined as a subluxation or an immobilization of the occipital bone upon the atlas in any part of the movement of head-turning. The lesion is named according to the side toward which the head turns, occiput rotated to the right or occiput rotated to the left. The axis of motion is an almost vertical one projecting upward from the articulation of the dens with the transverse ligament.

The lesion is produced by muscular contracture, as an example of which may be mentioned torticollis; traumatism as by severe twisting or concussion; lack of balance in the contraction of opposing mucsles when strain occurs; proximity to infective processes from an extension of inflammation, and lastly from posture incident to securing relief from defective hearing, eyesight, or secondary to irritations in the cervical region.

CORRECTIVE MOVEMENTS

The principle of correction for a rotated occiput is rotation to the opposite side.

General Rules.—Contractured and thickened muscles and ligaments must be stretched and relaxed; atonic muscles must be given tone. When one side of the lesion is more closely restricted in motion than the other, a greater amount of attention should be given to that side.

Preliminary treatment may be given to the cervical region to secure relaxation of the long muscles reaching to the occiput and adjoining vertebræ. An attempt should be made to put the occipital articulations through the normal range of movement possible to them; in this way may ligamentous tissues be prepared for correction.

IV. Face-Turning Movement.—Let the patient, B, who has an occiput rotated to the right, lie supine upon the table with his head extending a few inches beyond its end against which O places his abdomen, a pillow interposed. O makes steady pressure against the top of B's head sufficient to maintain the head in the median plane of the body without support and without discomfort to the patient.

O places his left hand against B's left malar bone, the fingers pointing down, the middle finger applied to the adjacent edges of the tip of the mastoid process and the transverse process for the purpose of palpation to detect movement when it shall occur.

The right hand is placed beneath the occiput, grasping it to direct its movement in correction of that side of the lesion. The thumb is placed upon the adjacent surfaces of the ramus of the mandible and the transverse process to detect the beginning of motion upon that side.

O now adds slightly to the pressure on the top of B's head sufficient to lift the chin slightly and depress the vertex a little, the position one of slight extension. O carries B's chin to the right, turning the face somewhat in the same direction to bring the condyle into slight exaggeration of its immobilized position and also to give direction to the extension used to carry the right condyle forward, upward, and outward upon the underlying facet. Pressure is made against the left side of the face with the left hand while the right hand adds slight lifting force to the extension. O lifts the chin by increase of pressure in that direction, and, as the head is brought up to the limit of extension, the attempt at adjustment is made. Throughout the movement the top of the head is not to be carried from the median line.

If the correction were effected upon the right side the condyle should move forward to its normal position or beyond it at the moment extension is completed.

B's face is now turned gradually toward the left and the chin is carried to the left, back to the median line, the extension being held to that point. Then the top of B's head is carried into flexion by O's rising upon his toes while at the same time he depresses B's chin. The turning of the face and the carrying of the chin to the left continues until the chin has reached the limit of left lateral flexion and turning. Pressure is now directed downward upon both malar bones but especially upon the left in a line directed toward O's left knee which depresses B's chin strongly. O rises a little more upon his toes which carries the vertex higher. At this moment the left condyle should move backward, downward, and inward upon the underlying facet of the atlas. The palpating finger will detect this movement when it occurs.

The flexion is maintained while the chin is being carried back to the median line and the face turned to the right until the median plane is reached, at which time O sinks back upon his feet, at the same time lowering the top of B's head, elevating his chin, until the positions O and B hold are the same as those at the beginning of the corrective movement. The movement in its entirety should be repeated from five to ten times at each treatment.

If one side has a limited amount of movement and the other side is quite restricted, that half of the movement which applies to the restricted side should be repeated several times. It is often a simple matter to adjust the articulation which manifests slight mobility. As soon as it is apparent that correction of one part of the double lesion has been secured, the attention should be given almost solely to the articulation remaining in lesion for it would be unnecessary and even mischievous to continue the movement as a whole. If one articulation is exceedingly difficult to adjust, after a reasonable number of trials, the top of the head may be moved from the median plane of the body and sidebent to the side opposite the condyle which has become immobilized in the position inward and backward upon the corresponding facet; when the lesion is an upward, outward, and forward subluxation of the condyle, the case may be helped by sidebending the head slightly to the same side.

UNILATERAL OCCIPITAL LESIONS

There are four of these lesions possible, an occiput anterior on the left or on the right; an occiput posterior on the left or on the right. They are traumatic lesions usually, and are corrected by the methods of adjustment for a rotated occiput with emphasis upon the part which corresponds to the position the occiput has become immobilized in. These lesions may be defined as follows:

An occiput unilaterally posterior on the right is a lesion in which the right occipito-atlantal articulation is immobilized in the position of rotation to the right upon a vertically oblique axis drawn through the left articular facet.

An occiput unilaterally anterior on the right is a lesion in which the right occipito-atlantal articulation is immobilized in the position of rotation to the left upon a vertically oblique axis drawn through the left articular facet.

It sometimes happens that a patient who had originally a bilaterally posterior or anterior occipital lesion has correction made of one articulation instead of both entering into the immobilization known as the posterior occiput or the anterior occiput. The condition that remains is an unilateral lesion. Palpation of both articulations through the relative positions of the transverse process with the ramus and mastoid, will establish the diagnosis. A considerable amount of deposit may be found upon the side immobilized, a manifestation of the inflammatory sequences following upon the causative traumatism.

DIFFERENTIAL DIAGNOSIS

Since restricted motion is the characteristic of every lesion, differential diagnosis among lesions of the same articulation must be made by the presence of distinctive signs. An anterior occiput is easily differentiated from a posterior occiput for in the former there is a separation of the ramus from the transverse process while in the posterior occiput the ramus and transverse process are approximated. Both show the same distances vertically considered between the tip of the mastoid and the lateral edge of the transverse process while the characteristic sign of the lateral occiput is that the tip of one mastoid is approximated vertically and almost in the same vertical plane with the lateral border of the transverse process while the tip of the other mastoid process is separated in a vertical line from the transverse process and it projects beyond a plane erected vertically from the lateral border of the transverse process. Both mastoids are, however, equidistant from the rami of the mandible, a sign which differentiates the lateral occiput from some cases of a rotated occipital lesion.

The styloid process is sometimes mistaken for the transverse process when the patient has exceedingly small transverse processes. Careful palpation for the size and shape of the process should help to differentiate it from the transverse.

Paramastoid processes[1] are comparatively uncommon but when they are present upon both sides the diagnosis has often been mistaken for an ankylosed occipito-atlantal case. They may occur upon one side only; they are always placed posterior to the true mastoid processes and spring from the jugular processes of the occipital bone.

IN CONCLUSION

Treatment of occipital lesions must be carefully administered. The error of students and physicians is the use of too much pressure

1. Dwight Museum of Harvard University has at least three skulls showing the paramastoid processes. The entire osteological collection is valuable but the present encumbent of the office of curator is an old man and discourteous to scientific investigators from other schools of practice, offering a sharp contrast to the treatment accorded the author and other physicians by Wistar Institute in Philadelphia, The Royal College of Physicians and Surgeons, London, the Musee d'Ecole de Medicine, Paris, and other museums in this country and Europe.

against the top of the head or in movements through large arcs. Failure to adjust lesions of these articulations should be followed by a second trial using just as little force as possible. Rough treatment of cervical muscles in the nature of heavy massage must be interdicted, for dull, heavy aching is the usual consequence of such work.

Re-examination should be made at the beginning of each professional visit so that the possibility of over-correction will be avoided. Where faulty habit has been a causal factor in the formation of the lesion, then a small amount of over-correction is to be permitted but in cases of lesions which may progress to another type, as for example when a bilaterally posterior occiput is over-corrected upon one side and causes a rotated lesion, over-correction is almost malpractice on the part of the physician.

The planes of the articulating surfaces must be kept continually in mind in analyzing the modes of lesion production and correction. It should be unnecessary to state that the greatest skill is requisite for the adjustment of occipital lesions.

LESIONS OF THE ATLAS

The atlanto-axial articulations are the most freely movable of the vertebral joints. The characteristic movement between these two bones is rotation about the dens of the epistropheus as a pivot in a plane which is nearly horizontal. The arthrodial joints are formed between the inferior articular facets of the atlas and the superior articular facets of the epistropheus. These articular surfaces are covered with hyaline cartilage which is much thicker in the centre than at the circumference, another cause of increased mobility. It is believed that in the erect position the curved surfaces of the cartilaginous covering of the facets are in contact only and that the head is held erect by the action of opposed muscles.[1]

Flexion, extension, and sidebending also take place in the atlanto-axial joints but the last is always accompanied by rotation as a secondary movement just as rotation is accompanied by sidebending, due to the inclination of the superior articular sur-

1. See Morris, ibid., p. 222, paragraph 8, and p. 224, paragraph 2.

faces of the axis, which slope outward and backward. There is a certain amount of lateral gliding in the atlanto-dental articulation, so that when the atlas rotates to the right, it turns upon the dens, glides laterally and carries the greatest width of the atlantal mass which lies external to the articular facets, superior and inferior, to the right downward and backward; on the left carries the corresponding mass to the right upward and inward, bringing it closer to the central articulation and thereby elevating the left side of the head and depressing the right side. It is by this means that the crown of the head is brought to the horizontal after the production of a rotated occipital or lateral occipital lesion. A right lateral occiput, produced in left sidebending, depresses the left side of the head. A right lateral or rotated atlas bringing the greatest amount of height upon the left side of the atlanto-axial articulation closer to central axis and the median line, elevates the left side of the head and restores the crown of the head to the horizontal. Such a lesion of the atlas is a counterbalancing or secondary lesion having for its purpose the restoration of erectness to the head.

Immobilization of the atlanto-axial articulations is rare and is subsequent upon inflammation usually as the result of traumatism. Arthritis often invades these joints with the same characteristic sign of the primary atlanto-axial lesion, restricted motion.

The lesions of the atlas as classified by the terminology committee of the American Osteopathic Association, are three, as follows:

A lateral atlas is a lesion in which the atlanto-axial articulations are immobilized in the position of sidebending-rotation.

A rotated atlas is a lesion in which the atlanto-axial articulations are immobilized in the position of rotation-sidebending.

An extension lesion of the atlas is a lesion in which the atlanto-dental articulation is immobilized in the position of extension or upward gliding of the atlantal facet upon the dental facet. It is an unusual lesion, more often secondary in character. Often in cases of long-standing the dens of the epistropheus gradually increases in height with a corresponding elongation of its articular facet. In this lesion, the inferior articular facets of the atlas glide upward and forward upon the superior articular facets of the axis.

The lateral atlas lesions are named right or left according to the side upon which there is greater lateral prominence of the transverse process of the atlas. The rotated atlas lesions are named according to the side upon which the atlantal articular facet has rotated backward.

EXPERIMENTAL PALPATION, U.—Let the subject, B, who is assumed to have a lateral atlas lesion upon the right, sit upon a stool while O stands behind. O places the palmar surfaces of his index fingers against the lateral borders of the transverse processes of the axis to compare them with the overhanging transverse processes of the atlas. If a right lateral atlas lesion is present, the transverse process of the atlas on the right will extend laterally much beyond the same process of the axis, and the lateral border of the left atlantal transverse process will be in the same vertical line with the lateral border of the left axial transverse process. The patient is instructed to bend the head to the right and to the left, whereupon no change in the relative positions of the processes under palpation takes place, and the diagnosis is confirmed.

The diagnosis of a right lateral atlas lesion is established by the presence of the following signs:

1. Restricted motion.
2. Marked projection of the lateral border of the right transverse process over the corresponding process of the axis.
3. The approximation vertically of the lateral borders of the left transverse processes of the atlas and axis.
4. The presence of a counterbalancing lesion of the occiput.

THE PRINCIPLE OF CORRECTION FOR A LATERAL OR ROTATED ATLAS LESION IS SIDEBENDING TO THE SAME SIDE AS, OR ROTATION TO THE OPPOSITE SIDE FROM, THE LESION.

GENERAL RULES.—ANY OPERATIVE MOVEMENT WHICH WILL ADJUST AN OCCIPUT LATERAL TO THE RIGHT WILL ADJUST AN ATLAS TO THE RIGHT; ANY OPERATIVE MOVEMENT WHICH WILL ADJUST AN OCCIPUT ROTATED TO THE RIGHT WILL ADJUST AN ATLAS ROTATED TO THE LEFT, WITH THE ADDITION OF THE ESTABLISHMENT OF THE FIXED POINT AGAINST THE SIDE OF THE AXIS TOWARD WHICH MOVEMENT IS MADE, IN EACH LESION.

When these lesions occur as counterbalancing lesions to occipito-atlantal lesions, it is always necessary to adjust the occipital lesion first; when the atlas lesion is primary, it may be necessary to follow its adjustment with correction of the counterbalancing occipital lesion. There are scarcely any clinical reports extant of these cases but osteological specimens[1], chief of which may be mentioned those at Wistar Institute, confirm the few case histories obtainable.

1. The author has had in her possession during the past year one of the most valuable of these specimens, belonging to the private collection of Dr. Raymond S. Ward, of New York City. It is primarily a specimen of a lateral occiput with a secondary lateral atlas in which secondary changes in the bone formation have taken place. When the science of vertebral osteology shall have attained its proper place as a branch of anthropology, there will not be lacking osteological proofs of every osseous lesion.

CHAPTER X.

CLAVICULAR AND OTHER LESIONS

The clavicle helps to form two joints, the sterno-costo-clavicular and the acromio-clavicular. Of both of these articulations[1] subluxation may occur. The sterno-costo-clavicular joint affords the only connection between the trunk and the upper extremity and it takes part therefore in all movements of the shoulder girdle and arm. The meniscus or articular disc is the essential element in the articulation, not only separating the articulating surfaces of the bones, but binding them together and affording attachment to the anterior and posterior sternoclavicular and interclavicular ligaments; by its fixation the clavicle is held to the sternum and prevented from over-riding the superior margin of the manubrium when it is elevated or depressed rotating about an antero-posterior axis.

EXPERIMENTAL PALPATION, V.—Let the subject, preferably a child of ten to twelve years of age, sit upon a stool, with shoulders bare. O stands behind the subject and reaching around with his left hand he places the thumb internal to the sternal end of the clavicle, the index finger at its upper border and the middle finger at the margins of the articulating surfaces of the clavicle, sternum, and disc anteriorly, to palpate for movement while the shoulder girdle is raised, circumducted, and depressed. O grasps the upper arm just above the elbow and carries it from in front upward, over, and backward. Just as the arm is started backward upon a return in the movement of circumduction, O notes that the sternal end of the clavicle rotates upon its long axis, and glides upward, so that it is slightly higher than its fellow of the opposite side. O then lowers B's arm to the side and notes that the clavicle returns to its normal position.

O then raises B's arm backward and upward and as the arm approaches an elevation above the shoulder, O may note that the clavicle rotates on its long axis inward, so that its upper border is slightly posterior to and lower than the upper border of the clavicle of the other side.

The lesions of the sterno-costo-clavicular articulations are termed depressed or elevated clavicles. They are defined:

---

1. See Marion E. Clark, ibid., p. 453, 454. Deaver, ibid., Vol. I, p. 221-224; Cunningham, ibid., p. 1444, 1445. Gray, ibid, p. 303.

A depressed clavicle is a lesion in which the sternal end of the clavicle has moved backward and downward, or it is an immobilization of the sterno-clavicular articulation in the position of rotation of the clavicle upon its long axis wherein the front border has moved upward.

An elevated clavicle is a lesion in which the sternal end of the clavicle has moved forward and upward, or it is an immobilization of the sterno-clavicular articulation in the position of rotation of the clavicle upon its long axis wherein the front border has moved downward.

These lesions are usually the result of strain or traumatism, falls upon the outstretched arm, the shoulder, or with the arm grasping an object to prevent falling. Of the symptoms which have been relieved by correction of the lesions, according to clinical records, the most prominent is vascular goitre; among the others relieved by correction of the lesions, according to clinical records, are pharyngeal and tonsillar congestions, headache, dyspnoea, dysphagia, and esophagismus.

CORRECTIVE MOVEMENTS

THE PRINCIPLE OF CORRECTION FOR A DEPRESSED CLAVICLE IS ROTATION ON ITS LONG AXIS FORWARD; FOR AN ELEVATED CLAVICLE, ROTATION BACKWARD AND DOWNWARD.

GENERAL RULES.—SINCE THE SHOULDER GIRDLE MOVES AS ONE BONE, THE REPLACEMENT MUST BE EFFECTED BY THE LEVERAGE OF THE UPPER EXTREMITY PRINCIPALLY, WITH PRESSURE AGAINST THE UPPER BORDER OF THE CLAVICLE TO ASSIST IN GIVING THE MOVABLE BONE A TURN IN THE RIGHT DIRECTION.

I. FORWARD AND UPWARD MOVEMENT.—Let the patient, B, who has a depressed right clavicle, sit upon a stool, with O standing behind him. O grasps B's right arm just above the elbow and carries it forward and upward as high as it will be carried without discomfort to B, and then backward slowly while at the same time with his left thumb against the upper and inner margin of the sternal end of the clavicle O presses in the effort to raise the inner end of the clavicle and rotates it outward and forward. At a certain point about midway between the upward position and the backward position at the level of the shoulder, the greatest amount of force is brought to bear upon the clavicle to adjust its lesion.

O returns B's arm to his side, and while holding the inner end of the clavicle in place, he asks B to rotate his shoulder girdle himself, sometimes with resistance placed upon the upper surface of the shoulder.

Many of these lesions are difficult to retain in adjustment for the ligaments of the articulation have become so relaxed that it is only after repeated adjustments that the integrity of the joint is secure.

II. BACKWARD AND UPWARD MOVEMENT.—Let the patient, B, who has an upward subluxation of the right sterno-clavicular joint, be seated upon a stool as in the last movement, with O in the same position, holding B's right arm in the same way. O places the thumb of his left hand in front of the inner end of B's right clavicle directing pressure against the bone to assist in rotating it backward and inward when O shall have brought B's arm to the position in circumduction backward, upward, forward, and downward, at which rotation of the clavicle along its longitudinal axis upward and backward shall have been accomplished. That point is commonly just before the elbow reaches the greatest height above the shoulder.

Lesions of the fifth and sixth cervical vertebral articulations should be adjusted before the clavicular lesions may be expected to remain corrected, for these lesions directly interfere with the nerve supply to the sterno-costo-clavicular joints.

The depressed lesion of the sterno-clavicular joint is the commoner of the two.

ACROMIO-CLAVICULAR LESIONS

The presence of the acromio-clavicular joint is a necessity if in shoulder movements the angle of the scapula shall lie against the thoracic wall and if the glenoid cavity of the scapula shall face the same way in every position, thereby putting upon the movement of the shoulder joint no restrictions. The movements of the acromio-clavicular joints are two, a gliding of the clavicle upon the acromion anteriorly and posteriorly and a rotation of the acromion upon the clavicle. Both movements are very slight in extent and difficult of palpation in any but the youthful individual who has little adipose tissue.

EXPERIMENTAL PALPATION, W.—Let the subject, B, be seated upon a stool, O standing behind him. O places the palmar surfaces of one or two fingers upon the upper surface of the outer extremity of the clavicle and the tip of the acromion process of the scapula. The eminence at the extremity of the clavicle will assist in locating the articulation. O grasps B's right arm above the elbow and raises it directly to the side until it is on a level with the shoulder-joint. No change in the relations of the articulating surfaces of the joint may be palpated. O then carries the arm straight backward and it may be observed that the clavicular extremity glides forward upon the acromion. O then turns B's arm in downward and backward rotation and the clavicular extremity becomes more prominent showing this movement rotates the scapular articulating surface downward and forward. He then returns the arm to the side.

O then repeats the raising of the arm and carries it up and over backward, which manifests at once a rotation of the scapular facet upward and backward.

The lesions of the acromio-clavicular articulation are those of elevation and depression. They occur rarely but because of the distressing symptoms following in their train, they are important to understand. They are usually caused by falls. The arm may have been thrown above the level of the shoulder. Sometimes a fall directly upon the shoulder will cause the lesion.

Pain is the most constant symptom of this lesion but because of the immobilization of the joint, in a position of normal movement, restricted movement characterizes the joint. The individual having the lesion finds it impossible to put on his coat, comb his hair, or reach into a hip-pocket.

CORRECTIVE MOVEMENTS

THE PRINCIPLES OF CORRECTION FOR ACROMIO-CLAVICULAR LESIONS ARE ROTATION OF THE SHOULDER UPWARD AND BACKWARD FOR AN ELEVATED CLAVICLE AND ROTATION UPWARD AND FORWARD FOR A DEPRESSED CLAVICLE.

GENERAL RULES.—IF THE LESION IS ONE OF SOME DURATION, IT IS OFTEN NECESSARY TO ATTEMPT MOVEMENT IN ALL DIRECTIONS BEFORE ADJUSTING THE LESION. DIRECT ADJUSTMENT IS NOT ALWAYS POSSIBLE, THEREFORE, THE CLAVICLE ITSELF SHOULD BE GUIDED INTO PLACE ACCOMPANIED BY ROTATION, ELEVATION, AND DEPRESSION OF THE SHOULDER IN TURN.

III. SHOULDER-RAISING MOVEMENT.—Let the patient, B, who has a depressed lesion of the right clavicular extremity, be seated upon a stool, with O standing behind him. O places the finger or thumb of his left hand in front of the outer third of the clavicle with the palmar surface of a finger palpating the articular surfaces of the joint. O then grasps B's right arm at the elbow or above, and carries the arm at right angles to the thorax laterally and then rotates it upward and forward meanwhile lifting by the left hand the clavicle into position. Three or four repetitions of the movement may be necessary to maintain the clavicle in adjustment.

IV. BACKWARD LIFTING MOVEMENT.—Let the patient, B, who has a backward and upward subluxation of the acromial end of the right clavicle, sit upon the end of the table, O standing to his right and behind him. O places his left hand over the shoulder, the thumb under the spine of the scapula to assist in lifting it, the fingers upon the prominent extremity of the clavicle to assist in guiding it back to its accustomed place in the articulation. O grasps B's right arm by the wrist, carries it backward in extension rotating it inward at the same time and gradually raising it by a vibratory movement[1] until it has been elevated to an angle of sixty or seventy degrees with the side of the thorax. Correction should be effected toward the conclusion of the movement.

The above movement may be varied by O's carrying B's forearm behind B's back after it has been raised about thirty degrees from the side, the left hand serving to guide the extremity of the clavicle into position. This movement[2] is used for the adjustment of a clavicle elevated at the acromial end.

PAINFUL SHOULDERS

In connection with the subject of lesions of the acromio-clavicular joint, a differential diagnosis of its chief symptom, pain in the shoulder, should be made for the reason that ordinarily such pains are classed as neuritis, displaced biceps tendon, rheumatism, neuralgia, and bursitis.[3] By far the larger number of cases of painful shoulders are due to bursitis usually of the subacromial bursa. The cause may be quite the same as would produce a subluxation of the acromio-clavicular joint, traumatism by falls, blows, and strains. In the acute stage the characteristic symptoms

1. Method preferred by Dr. John A. MacDonald of Boston.
2. Dr. Alex. F. McWilliams of Boston uses this method by preference.
3. See "Differential Diagnosis", by Richard C. Cabot, second edit., 1912, p. 325, 327, 330, 331, 338.

are pain about the joint, sensitiveness to pressure just below the acromial process and over the bicipital groove, when the arm hangs at the side. When the arm is abducted and rotated externally, limitation of motion is discovered on account of the extreme pain that results from compression of the bursa in these movements. At night the pain is worse. Relief is obtained by rest, anodyne applications, and elevation of the shoulder, as when the patient sits upon a stool in front of the physician, and the latter, resting his foot upon the stool beside the patient, places his knee in the axilla and thus elevates the shoulder. Grasping the arm near the elbow, with some slight traction downward, it may be stretched, which often assists in giving relief. The chronic form of bursitis may need surgical interference.[1]

There is a class of cases[2] which from slight injury, exposure to cold, or over-use with fatigue, manifest considerable pain and inconvenience not especially increased upon action. Careful examination should be made to exclude all the diseases which exhibit pain in the same region, as osteomyelitis, malignancy of bone, joint fringes, synovitis, acute infectious polyarthritis, and angina pectoris. Osteopathic examination will exclude subluxations of the clavicle at either end, of the first rib, of cervical or thoracic vertebræ. Contractions of the muscles of the shoulder are always present and yet the case does not warrant the designation of myalgia for the reason that use does not greatly increase the pain. These cases are amenable to osteopathic treatment through a restoration of circulation to the shoulder.

The treatment for this class of cases is palliative with the idea of putting the joint through the range of normal movement with especial attention to relaxation of the surrounding muscles by separating their origins from their insertions. An agreeable method is to rotate the shoulder affected and by gradual means approach circumduction.

---

1. See Ashhurst, ibid., p. 466, 467; Royal Whitman, ibid., p. 493-496.

2. Dr. Kendall L. Achorn in the "Clinical Department" of the Jour. of the A. O. A., Sept., 1914 and April, 1915, has gathered case reports with expression of opinion from some prominent osteopathists regarding the treatment of painful shoulders; among these may be mentioned Drs. George J. Helmer, George Tull, Normal B. Atty, and Ernest Proctor, who have cited cases in point with the above.

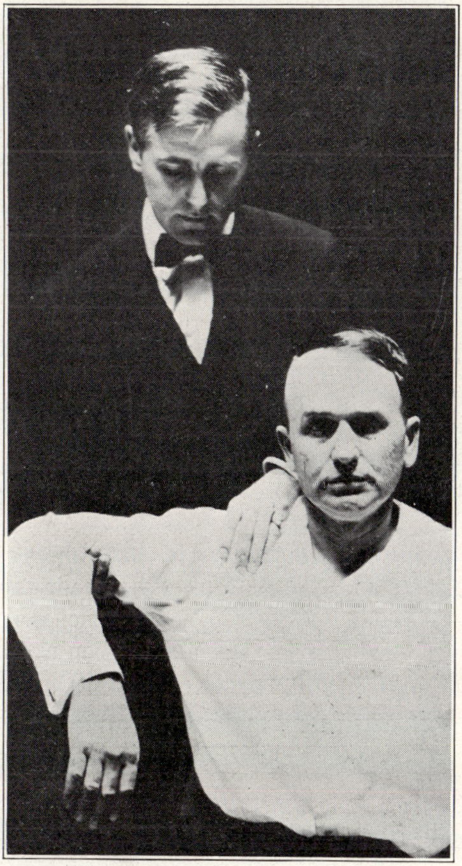

Fig. 82—Illustrating a method of taking hold of the upper arm and of the acromio-clavicular tissues in treatment of a painful shoulder.

VI. Arm-Circumducting Movement.—Ask the patient who is afflicted with a steady pain about the shoulder and much contraction of the muscular and ligamentous tissues, to sit upon a stool, O standing behind him. O grasps B's arm just above the elbow and beginning quite close to the side of the patient carries it in rotation and circumduction both forward and backward, gradually increasing the amount of circumduction, raising the arm to a constantly higher level but not to the extent that the arm is strained or fatigued. The movements must be slowly executed and gently given with perfect relaxation on the part of the patient. It may require six or ten treatments to overcome the condition, depending upon its severity and chronicity.

Acute brachial neuritis is a serious condition, demanding attention to the underlying causes with treatment of the same, especially to the correction of cervical lesions affecting the brachial nerve trunks, the upper thoracic lesions affecting the vaso-motor fibres supplying the area. Manipulative treatment of the arm is contraindicated, save when at the terminal ramifications there is evidence of atrophic conditions and then gentle measures locally applied with the purpose of increasing circulation are prescribed.

LESIONS OF THE MANDIBLE

The temporo-mandibular articulation is a complex one, consisting virtually of two joints, an upper and a lower, the former being formed by the meniscus and the anterior part of the mandibular fossa and adjacent glenoid ridge; the latter, by the meniscus and the condyle of the mandible. The movements of the lower jaw are compound, that which takes place in the upper joint consisting of a gliding forward slightly of the cartilage; in the lower joint, of a revolving of the condyle upon a transverse axis upward and forward or an alternate action of the two condyles, wherein the one which starts the movement not only revolves forward but also rotates upon a central vertical axis inward; upon its regression, the other advances; the movement of both schematically outlined would be represented by a figure 8 horizontally drawn. It has been called an oblique rotatory action.

EXPERIMENTAL PALPATION, X.—Let the subject, B, sit near the end of the table. O stands in front of him. B is instructed to open his mouth and then close his teeth without closing the lips. O notices whether or not the front teeth of the lower jaw and those of the upper meet exactly. O then moves behind B and places his fingers, palmar surfaces apposed, against both temporo-mandibular areas. B is then instructed to open and close his mouth. O may palpate the condyle as it moves forward and back. B is then given something to grind with his teeth and O observes the triturating movement, or alternate advance, rotation,

1. See Cunningham, ibid., p. 313; Gray, ibid., p. 279-281, 380; Frazer, ibid., p. 247, 250; Ashhurst, ibid., p. 392; Morris, ibid., p. 215-218, 342.

and return of each condyle. If the articulations are normal, no difference will be palpated between the two sides in each movement.

If B's teeth do not meet anteriorly, the lower ones showing that the mandible swerves to the right, when O palpates laterally, he will usually find that, upon the side away from which the jaw turns, the condyle, in depression of the jaw, moves more quickly and farther forward than upon the other side. Careful palpation through several movements will reveal the fact that motion in the left articulation shows less limitation than in the right articulation.

The temporo-mandibular lesion is a relaxation lesion with stretched pterygoid muscles, ligaments, and usually with hypermobility of the disc. Its most frequent cause is strain during the movement of trituration, through an attempt to bite down upon a hard object, the joint upon the side that is strained being in action, the other joint stationary. It may be due to the growth of a wisdom tooth unbalanced by the appearance of its fellow upon the opposite side. Frequently, through extension of an inflammation, such as otitis media, pharyngitis, parotitis, the joint may become hypermobile or upon the opposite side contracted leaving the bulk of mastication for one side, whereupon muscular unbalance results with the sequence of a relaxation lesion. When the meniscus is very loosely apposed to the glenoid fossa and ridge, a clicking sound may be heard whenever the individual eats, a source of great annoyance. Among the symptoms of which these patients have complained, according to clinical evidence, are neuralgia of any of the branches of the trigeminal nerve, tic douloureux, and headache.

CORRECTIVE MOVEMENTS

THE PRINCIPLE OF CORRECTION FOR A LESION OF THE TEMPORO-MANDIBULAR ARTICULATION IS RESISTANCE REPLACEMENT UPON THE SIDE IN RELAXATION AND PTERYGOID AND LIGAMENTOUS STRETCHING UPON THE SIDE IN CONTRACTION.

GENERAL RULES.—REPLACEMENT OF THE CARTILAGE AND CONDYLE UPON THE RELAXED SIDE MUST BE SECURED. BILATERAL RESISTANCE MUST BE OFFERED AGAINST MANDIBULAR DEPRESSION, PROTRUSION, AND RETRACTION.

III. CONDYLE REPLACING MOVEMENT.—Let B, the patient, be seated upon a stool, O standing behind him. If B has a relaxation lesion of the right temporo-mandibular articulation, O places the palm of his left hand against the left side of B's chin, grasping the chin so that he may push it to the righ . He then places the palmar surface of his right thumb in front of the right condyle of the mandible. B is asked to open his mouth, and then to close it while O assists in the replacement of the condyle by pressing against it with his thumb and pushing the mandible to the right with the left hand.

O then holds strongly against the jaw to resist its swerving to the left while B opens and closes his mouth several times. O then places the fingers of his left hand underneath the chin, the heel of the hand against the mental process. He asks B to open his mouth while he resists the movement with his fingers, and then instructs him to close his mouth, while O resists the closing with the heel of his hand. This movement is repeated several times at the conclusion of each treatment.

The time that is required to correct a lesion of these joints depends altogether upon the rapidity with which the atonic muscles and ligaments become normalized.

LESIONS OF THE HYOID

The hyoid bone is suspended under the mandible by muscles and ligamentous elastic tissues. It is connected with the larynx by four ligaments and the thyrohyoid muscle[1]. By irritation through surrounding and connecting tissues, it may be displaced upward or downward with contractured and shortened supporting tissues. Irritation is quickly manifest through the internal laryngeal nerve, which pierces the thyrohyoid membrane, and by it is communicated to other branches of the superior laryngeal nerve and by connecting filaments to other nerves.

The commoner symptoms arising from the displacement of this bone are coughing, tickling in the pharynx, and a sensation of constriction in the thyrohyoid region.

The lesion is of the nature of a muscular lesion and its adjustment is accomplished, after careful diagnosis to ascertain where the principle contractions are located, by a stretching of all contractions of ligamentous and muscular tissues, and with replacement of the hyoid in position. Resistance exercise may be given by asking the patient to swallow while the physician holds the

1. See Gray, ibid., p. 153, 388, 1167-1168, fig. 985 on p. 1170, 1175, 1006 last paragraph.

Morris. ibid., p. 501, fig. 974 on p. 1212, figures 980 and 981 on p. 1216, p. 1216, fig. 985 on p. 1219.

Cunningham, ibid., p. 1387, fig. 855 on p. 1075.

hyoid bone by its cornua. Vibratory relaxation, gently administered, is often helpful in relaxing the thyrohyoid membrane and the intrinsic ligaments and muscles of the larynx.

SPONDYLOLISTHESIS

One of the rare lesions which has been noted in medical literature is a subluxation of the fifth lumbar vertebra, or the fourth and fifth lumbar vertebræ, in extension upon the sacrum. The term for this lesion is spondylolisthesis, which means a slipping of a vertebra. When the lesion occurs early in life, before there has been complete osseous development of the parts of the lumbar vertebræ, there is exceedingly great deformity in the vertebræ taking part in this subluxation, in fact it may be a congenital malformation.

Acquired spondylolisthesis is the result of overstrain, injury, or weakness resulting in displacement from inability to manage superincumbent weight. In consequence of the change in equilibrium, secondary changes begin simultaneously above and below, with a resultant posterior sacral lesion and lessened pelvic inclination; above, one of two changes takes place, either the whole lumbar spine goes forward in lordosis or the fourth lumbar vertebra becomes lesioned in flexion and the spine above becomes straight. Diagnosis is made by palpation per rectum or vagina.

The symptoms are those which would naturally follow so marked a disturbance in balance, weakness and pain in the back, often radiating down the limbs, awkward carriage and gait, lowered resistance. It occurs more often in females than males. The change in the pelvis renders parturition exceedingly dangerous and the Caesarian section is indicated.

When there is deformity apparent, treatment may do little or nothing in the way of adjustment or correction. If, after X-radiance has shown the exact condition, there is a chance to change the relation of the articulating surfaces, the treatment would be that for any extension lesion coupled with treatment directed to the overcoming at the same time of all the secondary lesions, especially those of the sacro-iliac articulations.

Bibliography: Royal Whitman, ibid., p. 142-144.
"Practical Obstetrics," Grandin, Jarman, and Marx, 1909, p. 347.
Bradford and Lovett, 3d edit., 1907, p. 385-388.
"Handbook of Obstetrics," R. Cadwallader, 1908, p. 231-232.

CHAPTER XI.

SOFT TISSUE TECHNIQUE

The osteopathic physician recognizes that treatment of the soft tissues of the body is a necessity when a condition of stasis, interrupted nutrition, mechanical constriction, or malposition exists. Such treatment may be a complete system in itself and be applied successfully by those who have been specially trained. Sweden and Germany have had schools whose graduates were admirably fitted for handling these cases. Some persons there have been who from ignorance supposed that the school of osteopathic practice taught a system not unlike that of the foreign institutions. It should, however, be quite readily seen from what has gone before that while the osteopathic physician himself may use any or all methods of increasing the tone of soft parts, of removing detritus, etc., yet this represents by no means the central thought in his treatment. The osseous lesion is the basic foundation of the mechanics of osteopahty.

The engineer may oil the movable parts of his machine and feed it with fuel and water, but unless it has been adjusted, part to part, perfectly, he knows that it is illy equipped for any risks. The human being may be given food, drink, occupation, periods of rest, and soft tissue massage, but while vertebral subluxations remain, he is no better fitted to travel the road of life than the locomotive with a loose pin or worn nut. Dr. Orren Smith has in this connection offered an apt comparison: "Manipulation is the warm poultice of the nurse; adjustment is the keen knife of the surgeon."

Soft tissue work has certain well-defined therapeutic purposes, namely: stimulation; inhibition; equalization, referring to muscular unbalance; relaxation; reflex activity; preparation, in anticipation of mechanical replacement of subluxated units; palliation in acute conditions, and adjustment when used in relation to malpositions or ptosis. These will now be considered in greater detail.

Stimulation and inhibition are terms which have been used to describe the manner of manipulating the tissues of the body. Stimulation usually consists of a quick stroking or rotary massage. Inhibition consists of slow, steady pressures, often applied with stretching of the underlying or adjacent tissues.

The term stimulation has reference to mechanical excitation, when used osteopathically. It may or may not coincide with the physiological meaning of the term. Inhibition, however, has little in accord with the use of the same word in nervous physiology. After the publication of the results of Sherrington's experiments, especially those in which he had been assisted by Alexander Forbes, the clinical evidence that had been collected by the founder of osteopathy and his early followers took more definite form, and certain well established facts may now be offered for laboratory proof:

A. The presence of definite centres, by which are meant areas at which stimulation may most speedily secure effect upon the final common efferent neuron.

B. The presence of secondary centres, points at which, following fatigue of the synapse from stimulation at a primary centre, excitation will promptly bring a response from an organ or tissue.

C. The production of vaso-motor reactions which assist in establishing immunity, through overcoming the persistence of conditions which invite infection and through changing the specific properties of the blood so that antibody formation is hastened and disease limited.

These experiments also explain certain phenomena observed by practicians, as:

1. Long treatments often deplete the organism, bring no relief, and may be followed by increased severity of symptoms. The explanation is that excessive stimulation amounts to inhibition, since synapses have limited endurance, become fatigued, and cease to be capable of conduction.

2. Treatment which is not specifically directed to a correction of the existing condition but which by way of good measure is applied to both primary and secondary centres at the same time fails to have a beneficial effect. The cause of this failure to secure

results is that counterstimulation[1] of sufficient intensity causes the fields of dispersion to overlap and incoordination is the effect. Lack of coordination is the product of purposeless excitation.

3. The quick relief from infection which is obtained in patients who have had osteopathic treatment, when the acute condition is handled without drugs and by osteopathic therapeutic measures only, proves that the more a pathway is traveled, the less resistance it offers at the synapse. This also demonstrates that manual mechanics constitute what is truly a natural process for unlike the drug remedial agent,[2] it does avail in acute diseases regardless of its previous use in a tonic way or for chronic conditions.

4. A great many patients receive almost instant relief from a purposeful, well-directed treatment which lasts not longer than from three to five minutes. In explanation of this it should be stated that a single stimulus by association fibres may be relayed to the whole cord. As an instance of this may be cited those cases where adjustment of a spinal lesion brings almost immediate and perfect abatement of distressing symptoms. Cessation of excitation[3] may be expressed in inhibition. This may be offered as the foundation for Dr. A. T. Still's oft repeated dictum, "Find it; fix it; leave it alone."

V. Patients suffering from systemic diseases do not show immediate or noticeable response to specific adjustment or soft tissue treatment. The cause is general and recovery is slowly made. The cause lies in resistance at the synapse through the presence of toxins which result in increased resistance preventing stimulation of the final common neuron. Other causes operating in the same way are deficient local nutrition through interference with the blood supply, its volume, its quality, and deficient elimination of waste products. Changes in blood pressure markedly influence the condition of the synapse.

VI. Some patients will not respond to treatment administered by certain physicians. This may be called voluntary inhibition

1. Stimulation applied simultaneously to two areas.

2. The human body acquires an immunity to drugs, so that even increased or lethal doses show no appreciable effect upon the system.

3. As an example of this excitation may be given the spinal lesion which acts as an irritant.

for the patient consciously or unconsciously through the basal ganglia or cortex increases the resistance at the synapse. The reactive effects of cerebral inhibition are less under osteopathic therapy than that which employs drugs, for the drug acts as a toxin, often of virulence, in such patients.

There is such a wide difference in the manner of administering soft tissue treatment that in these pages the manner of its performance can only be suggested. That which is most commonly employed is directed to overcoming muscular unbalance. It is done, after the manner that has been discussed in these pages, by stretching the muscles, whenever leverage is available, through separating the origin and insertion of each muscle. By direct, so-called inhibitive pressure, steadily and firmly applied over the muscle mass, relaxation of contractions may be secured, and balance restored. By a series of small rotary movements across the muscle fibres, relaxation may be accomplished. The manner of doing these things has followed no hard and fast rules as with massage and mechano-therapy for the physician who applies such manipulations understands perfectly the tissue under his fingers and intelligently applies whatever he thinks necessary, taking into consideration each case as a separate entity. A preliminary course in massage would avail a student nothing, in fact it might be a decided disadvantage by leading to routinism in treatment. The touch of the physician should always be used with a diagnostic purpose. If he gives manual relaxation, it should be applied with constant observation, so that physiological limitations will be strictly obeyed.

The circulation to various parts may be improved, either through increasing anabolism or katabolism. The treatment of the liver is a marked example of this. The patient is placed in one of three positions for direct manipulation of the liver. When he lies supine, with his knees flexed, the physician, standing at his left, places his left hand under the angles of the right seventh to tenth ribs, his right hand upon the chondral ends of the same ribs a little external to their extremities. By simultaneously raising up with the left hand and compressing with the right hand and then releasing the pressures quickly, the liver is given a slight shock which stimulates the blood and biliary circulation.

Another method, which has been suggested by figure 72, page 180, is administered with the patient lying upon the left side, the physician standing behind the patient, who is asked to reach with his right hand across the physician's back and grasp his right shoulder. The ribs of the right side are all elevated by the physician's moving back in extension upon the patient's right shoulder. The hands are placed in the same position as in the movement above. The patient may be instructed to take a full breath and as he exhales, the physician bends over his thorax placing compression by his chest against its lateral wall and with his hands compression anteriorly and posteriorly. A quick release is made following the close of expiration.

A favorite method with many osteopathists is to treat the liver with the patient in the knee-chest position in practically the same way with additional lifting upward if there is any visceral ptosis present.

In tonsillar and pharyngeal congestions, drainage may be promoted by relaxation of the tissues above the area of the hyoid bone and in the infra-mandibular region. The movements given are usually downward in direction.

The eye is an organ helped often by soft tissue treatment, which is administered by gentle tapping upon a finger resting over the eye-ball or by slow and gentle compression of the eye-ball. A stroking of the upper eyelid from the lachrymal gland toward the inner canthus, if it is done with exceedingly gentle movement, is soothing and palliative in conjunctival inflammations.

Gynecological massage is a subject that has been so thoroughly covered by the texts upon the subject that reference here is unnecessary beyond the statement that it is the treatment par excellence for non-surgical cases.

In acute cases, due to the wide variance in etiology and pathology, it would be futile to attempt a description of the methods employed. Such treatment is better discussed in a text upon practice.

Visceral ptosis, when its diagnosis has been established, comes especially within the province of the osteopathist, who first of all removes vertebral and costal lesions, corrects postural defects, and lastly replaces viscera in their normal locations and brings tone to supporting connective tissues.[1] This is not done by a general kneading of the abdominal contents, but by lifting the viscera, with the patient in the knee-chest or Trendelenburg position. The palmar surfaces of the fingers should be insinuated in among the tissues until the organ that shows the greatest deviation from normality is found and then lifted to its normal place in the abdomen. This applies particularly to the different parts of the colon, the stomach, and the kidneys. The patient must be taught the value of exercise for the abdominal muscles, especially breathing exercises of the abdominal type with expulsive exhalations. These exercises should be practiced before the physician so that there shall be no misunderstanding about the manner of taking them. The patient must also learn to contract slowly the abdominal muscles while lying supine or in either of the positions suggested above. He may even be taught to massage his own intestines, carefully raising them up toward the thorax, as a daily exercise.

The manner of doing abdominal work must be touched upon. Dr. A. T. Still[2] has recently said, "Keep the points of your fingers out of all abdomens because if you do not you will bruise a kidney, an ureter, a spleen, the peritoneum, the omentum, or the liver, all of which are liable to injury by rough handling." Again[3] he says, "You must not hurt your patients while you are treating them. My observation has been that he who hurts his patient shows his lack of skill."

Abdominal treatment for the replacing of viscera and increasing the activity of the liver is a part of what has been termed the general treatment, whose expressed purpose is tonic effect given to the entire system. This does not mean to the discriminating osteopath soft tissue manipulation of the entire body, but rather a spinal treatment in the nature of normal movements given to vertebral articulation, to the occipito-atlantal joints, and to the sacro-iliac articulations. The argument for such a plan of treatment is that since a change of circulation is beneficial to all tis-

1. See Dr. C. P. McConnell's article in the Jour. of the A. O. A., June, 1912, p. 1159.

2. A. T. Still, "Research and Practice", p. 209.

3. Same text, p. 88.

sues, nowhere in the system would a better circulation avail more than about the central nervous system. Spinal movements are those which most quickly change the cordal circulation. The treatment of the sacro-iliac articulations has for its purpose relief from the strain incident to the static positions of the body throughout the waking hours.

It is not every patient who can take a general treatment and the physician needs to exercise judgment in selecting those who may with impunity receive what they ask for, the general tonic treatment. It has its danger for the physician, when too often repeated, of routinism, which has been the bane of medical therapy since the beginning. The medical practitioner who always prescribes the same drugs for every case that presents the same symptoms soon becomes mired in the ruts of habit. The perfection of the art of diagnosis means nothing to him, improved methods of therapeutic practice pass him by unnoticed or at best arouse his antagonism. The only danger which besets the osteopathic physician is the alluring sameness of general treatment, leading to mental inertia and physical depletion.

It might be said, **in conclusion,** that osteopathy stands for increased tissue fortification, chemical resistance, high-grade bodily efficiency, health. If it would seem that too much emphasis has herein been placed upon the osseous lesion and its adjustment, it may be pointed out that no other system of medicine embraces this peculiar form of diagnosis or mechanistic principle of correction and while the physician of the osteopathic school is counted a skilled exponent of anatomic adjustment of part to part, yet he is in every sense a true physician, side by side with physicians of all other schools waging the battle with disease, be it physical, mental, or moral. We believe that when Andrew Taylor Still gave to the world the principle that the rule of the artery is absolute he laid the cornerstone of the healing art and that when the superstructure of the days to come shall be reared, it will rest upon the anatomic foundation demonstrated by the constructive methods of the science of osteopathy.

ADDENDA

EXAMINATION OF A PATIENT.—The student who has completed the study of corrective movements naturally asks the question, "What is the best approved method of examining a patient to discover his lesions?" There is a preferred method and for the assistance of the student it is here offered in the order that has been followed by the best osteopathists:

INDEX